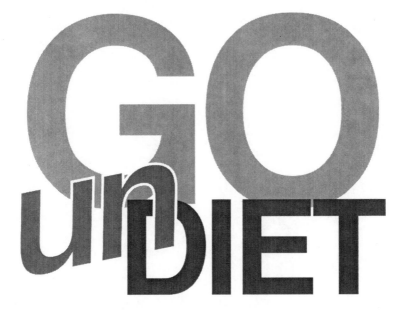

GO unDIET

50 Small Actions for Lasting Weight Loss

Gloria Tsang, RD

ISBN 978-0-9832167-9-7

First Edition: June 2011

The information in this book should not be used for diagnosing or treating any health problems. Not all diet plans suit everyone. You should always consult a trained healthcare professional or a registered dietitian before starting a diet. The author and publisher disclaim any liability arising directly or indirectly from the use of this book.

HealthCastle® and Go UnDiet™ are trademarks of HealthCastle Nutrition.

Trade names and trademarks mentioned in this book are used in an editorial fashion only and no infringement is intended.

To The Loves of My Life
Ian, Amy, Alan, and Polly

Table of Contents

Introduction   ix

Chapter 1: Forget About Breakthroughs;
    Take Small Steps Now   1

Chapter 2: Learn Which Packaged Foods to Avoid   11

Chapter 3: Re-learn Your Fats   31

Chapter 4: Don't Be Fooled by a High-Fiber Claim   48

Chapter 5: You Don't Need to be Vegan to Eat Healthy   65

Chapter 6: Study Your Drinks   84

Chapter 7: Add Color and Carbs to Your Plate   99

Chapter 8: Watch Out for the Extras   118

Chapter 9: Do Your Homework Before You Invest in
    Your Health   131

Chapter 10: Look Beyond Calories   148

Chapter 11: Putting It All Together   158

Appendices   164

About Gloria   177

Endnotes   179

Index   189

Acknowledgements

I would never have been able to complete this book without the love of my husband, Ian Lee. You gave me unconditional support and courage. Eleven years ago, you gave me a card that said "Walk the Untraveled Path," which I've kept on my desktop until this day. Thank you for listening to my ideas in the middle of many nights, and truly knowing what I'm made of.

To my parents, Alan and Polly Tsang: Thank you for being my role models and teaching me to persevere. I grew up never giving up, and believing that sky is the only limit.

To my closest friends, Sofia Layarda, Kei Lau, and Janice Chan: I have been bouncing my book idea off you for the past four years. Thank you for your no-nonsense, honest feedback; you've helped me fine-tune my untamed ideas.

To my research assistants, Sofia Layarda, MPH, RD; Jessica Hookham, RD; and Tracey Johnston: Without your help, I couldn't have put together all the scientific findings and background information in such orderly fashion. And to my editor, Christina Newberry: You've transformed my ideas into a joyful read!

To my long-time mentor, Patricia Chuey, RD: Your entrepreneurial spirit taught me that I could create a career for myself.

And thank you to all my colleagues and friends who offered help and feedback in my publishing journey: Judy Thomson;

Heather Jones, RD; Janis Donnaud; Nancy Clark, MS, RD; Janice Bissex, MS, RD; Joanne Lichten, PHD, RD; Brenda Ponichtera, RD; Julie Negrin, MS, CN; and John Chow.

And last but not least, to all my staff and partners: Owennie Lee, RD; Sejal Dave, MS, RD/LD, CDE; Beth Ehrensberger, MPH, RD; Keeley Drotz, RD, CD; Leah Perrier, RD; Elizabeth Daeninck, MS, RD; Andry Layarda; Peter de Rama; Silvia Kumala; Jessica Chen; Ann Carlsen; Karen Mori; William Cadman; and 1106 Design: Thank you for supporting my vision on HealthCastle.com and believing in me. Without you, I couldn't have furthered my passion—spreading the goodness of nutrition.

Introduction

I wrote this book for my website readers.

I would never have thought of writing this book if not for the requests of my readers on HealthCastle.com. I'm blessed that I have had so much support from my readers over the years—some even dating back to the late-90s, when I first started writing about my father's cancer journey. When I was in the family waiting room, waiting for my father during his daily radiation treatments, someone would often ask me about cancer treatment eating tips. I thought to myself, "I should put all the knowledge and experience I have about cancer nutrition on a website, so other families in the same boat can access this information." This was how HealthCastle.com came about in 1997.

Little did I know that my own personal hobby site could grow into the largest online nutrition network. In 2010, HealthCastle. com had 7.5 million readers. In the past five years, I have constantly received emails from readers and agents, asking me to write a book. To be honest, I was resistant! A diet book? I thought: I'm against dieting! I'm against following a diet! How could I write a diet book? I pondered the book-writing idea for two years. Then, one day in 2008, the idea of UnDieting came to me.

The very term "diet" has become taboo, because people now understand that diet plans don't work and may even be unhealthy.

Many diet plans encourage readers to tune out and disengage from making their own decisions. They sell a promise—a promise to lose x pounds if readers strictly follow the plan for x days. But you know that a rigid meal plan is hard to fit into a busy lifestyle—and that even if it works, a 14-day meal plan only creates results for 14 days. Instead of teaching dependence on charts and plans, this book teaches you how to take back control of your food and nutrition choices, allowing you to make small changes at your own pace and create dramatic change—without starvation—that results in real, healthy weight loss that lasts for the long term. It's not a diet—it's the UnDiet.

This book is a no-gimmick guide to help you stop the pendulum of weight loss and weight gain with 50 small actions that will change your diet and weight without the rigidity of a diet plan. Instead of zeroing in on just one nutrient or element of dieting (low carb, low fat, high fiber, etc.), this book empowers you to reclaim your health through small, achievable steps that last. By implementing one of the book's 50 simple Go UnDiet Actions every week, you make major changes over time without a sense of loss or sacrifice.

Let's start UnDieting now.

And get healthy one step at a time.

Forget About Breakthroughs; Take Small Steps Now

You've probably picked up this book because you're suffering from diet fatigue. The conflicting information that constantly bombards you—high carb versus low carb, low fat versus low sugar, high glycemic load versus low glycemic load, refined carbohydrate versus complex carbohydrate, and on and on—may have left you confused, frustrated, and searching for something better. Instead of another miracle diet plan, you just want something that works—a way to lose weight for good by making small changes in your eating habits that deliver big results that last for the long term.

I believe in science, but I'm also a believer in common sense. Scientific data tells me what can theoretically be achieved. It gives me a good ballpark estimate of what most people can do. But data isn't personal. It's entirely objective, and removes any ounce of human touch. What other people can do doesn't necessarily translate into what you can do. That's why this book is built around common sense. Before giving you any tip or Go UnDiet Action, I always ask, "Does it make sense?" and I encourage you to do

1

the same. You can only accomplish what makes sense to you, no matter what the science says. So before you try to implement any weight loss strategy, always ask yourself that one key question: "Does it make sense?"

Why Your Previous Dieting Flings Have Failed
They Sell a Promise, Not a Plan

Traditional diet plans encourage you to tune out and disengage from making your own eating decisions. They sell a promise—a promise to lose x pounds if you strictly follow the plan for x days. And it's true that you might lose the weight that they promise. But most diet books only give you a 14- or 28-day meal plan. So what happens when the 14 or 28 days are up? You could go back to Day 1 and start the plan again, but realistically, how many times can you do that? How are you supposed to follow the diet for the long term when you only know one specific meal plan that will work?

Diet books also encourage drastic cuts to your food intake so that you see quick results. Many of them encourage you to cut

---

UnDiet Q&A: What is a calorie?

A calorie (Cal or kcal) is a unit of measurement for the energy we take in from food and drinks, and the energy expenditure our bodies exert in order to perform an activity. An average adult female requires 1,800 to 2,400 calories per day, while an average adult male requires 2,200 to 3,000 calories per day.

Refer to Appendix A for further information on nutrition requirements.

To calculate your exact daily calorie requirement based on your age, gender, and activity level, use the free Calorie Calculator on my website http://www.healthcastle.com/calorie-requirement-calculator.shtml

---

500 calories or more a day. But just about everyone knows by now that cutting 500 calories is too drastic to last. An average woman needs about 2,000 calories per day. Cutting your intake by 500 calories to 1,500 calories will leave you hungry all the time! Let's face it—a 1,500-calorie diet is for eight-year-olds, not grown-ups.

You just don't need yet another "ground-breaking breakthrough" with a rigid meal plan and recipes that don't take your personal preferences into consideration, and that expects you to drastically cut your food intake to levels too low to keep you satisfied. Even if you can sustain yourself on a very low-calorie diet, your body will naturally adjust itself to slow down your metabolism.

You also don't need a set of so-called rules to follow that doesn't make any sense for your lifestyle or your body's needs. Diet plans not only tell you what to eat—they tell you when to eat, too! We've all heard that it's a good idea to eat small, frequent meals. Three meals per day plus one snack is the most common recommendation, but I've also heard five small meals per day and other variations. This is where common sense comes in. I just say to eat only if you're hungry. I eat three meals per day during the week, with no snacks. That's because I spend most of my time on weekdays working in front of my computer, and my activities are usually scheduled before dinner. I really don't feel hungry at all between meals, so it doesn't make any sense for me to snack in between. There's no reason to eat more often than your body tells you to just because it's in the rules of some diet plan.

 Go UnDiet Action #1: Start UnDieting
Stop starving yourself with an unreasonable diet plan or diet rules. Get ready to implement simple strategies that you can adopt for the rest of your life.

Get Healthy One Step at a Time

Most people want to eat better than they do—but exactly how to "eat healthy" can sometimes be an overwhelming question. It's easy to get caught up in trying to reach the absolute ideal. But if you try to do everything at once and achieve too much too soon, you're sure to be overwhelmed.

The Atkins diet, popular in the '90s, for example, has a list of allowed foods and a list of forbidden foods for phase one of the diet. Juice, caffeine, and alcohol are not allowed, along with a list of foods so long that you simply can't make it through phase one without constantly referring to the allowed and forbidden lists to check everything you plan on eating. The South Beach diet has a similarly restrictive phase one, with no grains, fruit, or alcohol. Yes, you may lose weight by implementing so many changes and severely restricting your foods, but you will gain all the weight back when you add these foods back into your diet.

No wonder diet plans can seem a little overwhelming. The problem is that once you start feeling overwhelmed, it's really easy to give up, and once you give up, it's very hard to get back on track. Instead of putting yourself through that painful cycle, why not aim for achievable progress by making one small change at a time? In the end, you will reach that healthy eating ideal, but you'll do it in a way that makes sense to you and allows you to maintain your healthy eating strategies for the long term.

 Go UnDiet Action #2: Start one change per week. This book gives you 45 Go UnDiet actions after this chapter. A life-changing habit usually takes time to establish, so please do not try all of these actions at once. Remember, temporary measures only result in temporary results. Only life-long habits will give you long-term results. Just try one action per week and tackle one obstacle at a time. If it takes longer than a week, let it be. Once you're comfortable with that action, add another.

What's Your Priority?

Ask yourself a tough question: What's your priority? People always tell me that they "want to lose weight," or "want to eat healthy," or "want to lower cholesterol." Do you notice something interesting about those statements? They all use the word "want." But it's not really about what you want. It's about what you can do, and what you're willing to do.

You may have great intentions when you set yourself the goal to lose 5 pounds in a month. But how good is that as a goal if you don't know how you're going to get there? You may hit that goal, or you may not. That's because your goal was really more of a want—and it completely lacked any plan of action.

 Go UnDiet Action #3: Start doing it.
Abstract goals like "lose 10 pounds by summer" don't mean much. So set an action goal for this week: "I'll do this one thing this week and stick with it." Then evaluate after a week to see how well you've met your action goal, and what results you've achieved.

Face Your Obstacles (and Excuses)

This book guides you along a flexible path to eating healthy, but you need to be in control of your own health. This is not a typical diet book. I won't encourage you to disengage from making your own health decisions, and I won't ask you to blindly follow a meal plan. In fact, I have no meal plans for you to follow! Instead, I want you to be able to assess your own habits and behaviors. Have you ever said any of the following?

- I don't have time to cook.

- I don't like to cook.

- I'm too tired to cook.

- I don't have time to eat breakfast.

- I don't like vegetables.

- I don't have time to grocery shop.

- I overeat at social gatherings, but that's okay. It doesn't happen all the time.

- I can't resist snacks, but that's okay. Everything in moderation, right?

- Yes, I'm overweight, but I'm healthy.

If so, it's time to stop making excuses and start putting your money (and time) where your mouth is. You can't achieve your health goals if you don't put healthy eating high on your priority list, and that means that you will have to do some cooking and shopping and, yes, eat some vegetables.

As you start to implement the actions in this book, you may hit snags or face temptation to go back to your old ways. You're going to need to put the old excuses away and start using problem-solving techniques to move forward instead of back. In the last section, I asked you to set an action goal and stick to it for a week. Now's the time to evaluate. Can you stick to that action this week? Have you come across any obstacles preventing you from doing it? Will you be able to overcome those same obstacles if you face them again in the future? If not, can you make some kind of compromise? How you decide to solve your own obstacles and compromises is entirely up to you, as long as you remember: No excuses!

 Go UnDiet Action #4: Start using problem-solving techniques.
You are the boss of your own body and health, so if you encounter obstacles, you need to figure out the best way to compromise, recalibrate, and get back on track.

It's Kick-Off Week

By now you should be starting to get a sense of what the Go UnDiet program will be like. But before you dive into Chapter 2, I'd like you to start with a kick-off week. The purpose of this week is to get you ready to start making the changes you'll read about through the rest of this book. For this week, I want you to start this: Keep a food journal.

Keep a Food Journal

Writing down what you've eaten is a powerful way to make yourself accountable for your own food decisions. In fact, studies have shown that people who keep food journals lose twice as much weight as those who don't.[1] That's probably because keeping a food journal makes you think more about the food you're eating, and helps keep you accountable to yourself.

Write down the time, the food, and the portion size each time you eat. Don't just write down meals—write down everything, including snacks and drinks, for a full week. And don't forget about condiments, like butter on toast or sugar in tea.

You may think that food journaling sounds awfully tedious, and that you can just keep a mental record of what you've eaten each day. I can only say that you won't have a truly accurate picture of what you've consumed until you have a truly accurate record. You can keep it simple by just writing things down in a notebook, or use an online tool like the one at LiveStrong.com, which also has a mobile app to help you journal on the go.

Keeping a food journal is meant to get you interested in what's in your food, and be conscious of what you're putting in your mouth. I'm not going to tell you what to eat. Instead, I am going to teach you how to identify your own trouble hotspots. After keeping your food journal for a week, take a look back and look for patterns, like:

- What's your biggest meal of the day?

- Do you prowl for an afternoon snack two or three hours after lunch?

- How many sweetened drinks do you have on an average day?

- What snacks do you eat on the weekends?

- How often do you pick up fast food?

And how honest were you with yourself? Did you ever purposely skip an entry because you knew the food was junk? Keeping and evaluating your own food journal is really a self-discovery process. You may find that for the first time, you realize how many little "extras" you consume during the day that add up to big calories that can challenge your weight loss goals.

After keeping a food journal for a week, it may just become a habit. You can keep doing this throughout the Go UnDiet program if you feel it is contributing to your success.

Get Moving

Another easy way to create a negative calorie balance is to get moving every day. No foods can help you burn calories; only physical activities can. For a 150-pound person, 20 to 25 minutes of fun activities can easily burn 200 calories! Go swimming, take your dog for a brisk walk, take a dance lesson, ice-skate around the rink, jump rope, get a racket to play a game, or take a spin at the park. Any of these activities can be enjoyed with a partner or your kids, so plan it into your day!

 Go UnDiet Action #5: Start your new life with a kick-off week.

Before you dive into the rest of the book, take this week to keep a food journal to get an accurate record of what you're really eating and find some fun activities to do every day!

Weight Gain = Calories In > Calories Out

If your daily energy need is 2,000 calories, but you eat 2,300 calories, you will have an excess 300 calories balance. Over time, you will gain weight. It takes about 3,500 excess calories to gain one pound of weight. By the same token, it takes 3,500 negative calories to lose one pound of weight.

So, how do you create a negative calorie balance? Like we just discussed, the best way is to simply add some daily activities. By burning more calories through physical activities, you are less pressured to eat less to compensate. Certainly, you can also eat less, but unfortunately, you may feel hungry if you eat less of the wrong food. In the following chapters, I'll help you identify certain high-calorie "villain" foods. You can cut them out of your diet and you won't even feel hungry.

5 Small Steps to UnDiet

This chapter's Go UnDiet Actions are all about setting yourself up for success as you work your way through the book. Take it slowly, work on one thing at a time, and ditch the excuses to establish the foundation of a successful life transformation with the Go UnDiet!

- ▶ **#1. Start UnDieting.** You're finished with yo-yo diets and starvation. Get ready to learn some real strategies for healthy weight loss that lasts.

- ▶ **#2. Start one change per week.** Implementing one action per week allows you to build up to major change without ever feeling overwhelmed or deprived.

- ▶ **#3. Start doing it.** Goals are great, but action is what makes things happen. Set an action-oriented goal, then follow through on it for a week.

- ▶ **#4. Start using problem-solving techniques.** If you go off-track or face an obstacle, look for ways to find your own solution.

- ▶ **#5. Start your new life with a kick-off week.** Keep a food journal to get an accurate picture of what you're really eating. This will get you ready to implement the steps in the rest of this book.

CHAPTER 2

Learn Which Packaged Foods to Avoid

We've all heard by now that we should try to avoid processed foods. But with the busy lifestyles we're all trying to navigate, sometimes it's just not possible for us to make every meal from scratch. So, are processed foods really the nutritional minefield they've recently been made out to be? Before we can answer this question, we need to take a look at how—and why—we ended up with so many processed foods in our grocery stores, and talk about the different kinds of processed foods you'll find there.

How We Got Here: The History of Processed Foods

What Exactly is Processed Food?

When you think about processed food, you probably picture things like hot dogs or snack products with a long list of unpronounceable ingredients. But the truth is it's only within the last 60 years or so that food processing has led to these food products that are so far removed from natural ingredients.

Originally, foods were processed to make them last longer. Think about your grandmother canning peaches or making strawberry jam. She was actually processing the peaches and strawberries so that you could get access to the nutritional value of the fruit even when peach trees and strawberry plants were not producing.

Even before canning and jam making became popular, meats were salted or smoked to keep them from spoiling, especially when no refrigeration was available. And, of course, most dairy products we consume today—even plain old milk—are processed, since they've been pasteurized both to extend shelf life and to slow microbial growth.

So, even if a food is not *highly* processed, like hot dogs or many snack foods, anything other than a whole, raw, natural food item (like an apple or a grain of wheat) is technically a processed food.

How Processed Foods Have Evolved

Things have changed a lot since those early days of processing food to preserve its shelf life and create year-long access to the nutrients of foods like fruits and vegetables that are only available at certain times of year. Since we all have fridges and freezers in our homes, and we can realistically buy imported peaches at any time of year, we don't need to use canned peaches as a substitute for fresh produce. And yet, supermarket shelves are stocked with canned fruits, and even canned pasta (which I cannot believe people actually eat!). Why? Food processing has gone to the extreme. Manufacturers no longer process food just to preserve its freshness.

Making it more appealing by adding artificial colors, reducing fat and sugar, enhancing texture and flavor, and so on are some of the reasons processing takes place. Many of these modern process-ing techniques are used to trick you into thinking the foods you're buying are better for you than they really are. So, let's take a look at what's really in some of those low-fat, sugar-free concoctions whose ingredients lists often read like the items needed for some kind of science experiment.

Highly Processed Foods: The "Low" Road
How Do They Reduce the Fat and Sugar in Foods?

Unlike foods that are simply processed, like your grandmother's canned peaches, for example, highly processed foods are pretty far removed from any recognizable whole food ingredient. Think about chicken nuggets. If you hadn't been exposed to chicken nuggets your whole life, would you be able to look at them and make any connection to a chicken? Ask yourself the same question when you think about foods that have low-fat or low-sugar claims. How do food manufacturers produce a food that looks and tastes so much like the original, but has less fat or sugar?

The simple fact is, of course, they add other ingredients to simulate the taste and texture of the fat or sugar that they remove. Often, this means the product is far enough removed from its original state that it can't even really be called the same product anymore. That's why, for example, you won't find low-fat mayonnaise or ice cream on store shelves. Instead, it's low-fat mayonnaise-style dressing and low-fat frozen dairy dessert.

So what do those low-fat and low-sugar claims really mean in terms of ingredients and impact on your body?

Low-Fat Does Not Mean Low-Calorie

When fat is removed from products to create low-fat versions, it is usually replaced with chemical-sounding additives and low-quality sugar. Since sugar is not calorie-free and provides half the calories fat does, this means that low-fat foods often have nearly as many calories as their full-fat counterparts—and it's calories, not just fat, that lead to weight gain.

Product	Reduced-Fat Version	Regular Version
Jif Peanut butter, 2 Tbsp	190 calories, 12 g fat	190 calories, 16 g fat
Nabisco Wheat Thins, 16 crackers	130 calories, 3.5 g fat	140 calories, 5 g fat
Nabisco Oreos cookies, 1 serving (1.2 oz.)	150 calories, 4.5 g fat	160 calories, 7 g fat
Nabisco Fig Newtons, 2 cookies	100 calories, 0 g fat	110 calories, 2 g fat
West Soy Soymilk, 1 cup	90 calories, 1.5 g fat	100 calories, 4.5 g fat
Quaker Natural Granola, ½ cup	183 calories, 2.6 g fat	210 calories, 6 g fat
Tostitos Tortilla Chips, 1 oz.	132 calories, 4.3 g fat	141 calories, 7.3 g fat

Table 1. Calories and fat in regular and reduced-fat foods

Plus, that low-fat claim has a way of playing tricks with our minds. Low-fat foods are often less satisfying to eat than their full-fat counterparts, so we need to eat more of them to get the same level of satisfaction. In fact, new research[2] suggests that "diet" foods may be satisfying at first, but they become less so over time. The researchers even suggest this may be one reason that so many of us find ourselves yo-yo dieting. We can live with reduced-fat and reduced-calorie foods at first, but after awhile we seem to crave the real thing.

Of course, while we are eating the low-fat versions, it's easy to convince ourselves that since there's less fat, it's okay to eat more. In the end, this can mean that you'll consume more calories eating low-fat cookies than you would if you chose the regular version.

Low-Sugar = Artificial Sweeteners

First, let's talk about what the various sugar claims you'll find on processed food packages actually mean. "Sugar-free" means that the product contains less than 0.5 g of sugar per serving. "Reduced sugar" means the product has at least 25% less sugar per serving than the reference food. And "no sugar added" means that no sugars were added during processing or packing (but the item might still contain natural sugars). Often, these reduced-sugar products are marketed as being better for kids. With childhood obesity and diabetes on the rise, you may think you're doing your kids a favor by limiting the sugar they consume. However, substituting artificial sweeteners for sugar is not a healthy way to cut sugar from your kids' diet—or your own.

When checking the ingredients list of a product, it can be hard to know which items are artificial sweeteners. Some common ones to keep an eye out for are sucralose, neotame, aspartame, acesulfame-potassium (Ace-K), and saccharin. More details on sweeteners are discussed in Chapter 8.

Instead of cutting down on sugar by using reduced-sugar products, look for foods that are naturally less sweet, but still satisfying. Or, instead of using a low-sugar version of a sweet cereal, cut sugar by mixing it half and half with an unsweetened whole grain cereal.

What About Low-Sodium?

In foods, sodium equals salt, and we all know that we have way too much salt in our diets. Indeed, we eat 50 percent more than the recommended level![3]

How much sodium should we eat?

2,300 mg (1 tsp) per day

The concern is due to the fact that consuming too much sodium can increase your risk of high blood pressure and other heart diseases.

Sodium is found in high quantities in many processed foods, including soup, canned vegetables and beans, frozen dinners, instant noodles, frozen pizza, sauces and dressings, pancake mix, processed meats, and crackers and cookies. Why is it so prevalent? Aside from taste and flavor, salt has a number of other important roles in processed food. It works as a preservative by preventing microbial growth, as early hunters discovered when they used salt to preserve their meat. It's also critical to the creation of fermented foods like pickles, cheese, and sauerkraut, as it enables the growth of the lactic acid bacteria needed to produce them. It enhances texture, for instance, by making cheese easier to shred and melt, and is used as an emulsifier in sauces and dressings. It helps leaven and condition dough used in baked goods. And, finally, just like home brining, salt improves tenderness in leaner meats. So leaner cuts of ham with lower fat usually have additional brine—which means higher sodium.

UnDiet Q&A: Are kosher salt and sea salt better than table salt?

Seasonings make food taste palatable, so it's unrealistic to shun all salt in home cooking. You can, however, reduce the amount of sodium you use by using different kinds of salt.

One teaspoon of iodized table salt contains over 2,300 mg of sodium. Kosher salt contains less sodium at 1,760 mg per teaspoon. Sea salt contains even less sodium: 1,570 mg per teaspoon.

Sometimes sodium appears on the ingredients list in modified forms, such as sodium chloride, sodium citrate, and sodium bicarbonate.

Since sodium is so prevalent in processed foods, it's important to limit it wherever possible. That means that a low-sodium claim can be a good thing!

 Go UnDiet Action #6: Un-low.
Highly processed foods (HPF) really do take the "low" road, promising lower fat and sugar contents, but replacing these ingredients with others that are usually just as bad for us. The only "low" claim that's really a good thing is low sodium.

Speaking of sodium, there is indeed another mineral that can counteract the damaging effect of sodium—and that is potassium.

Potassium can help lower blood pressure! This benefit was confirmed by the Third National Health and Nutritional Examination Survey (NHANES III). Data[4] on more than 17,000 adults indicated that adequate potassium intake from fruits and vegetables can lower blood pressure. Another study[5] also showed that people with a low sodium-to-potassium ratio (low sodium, high potassium) are less likely to suffer from a cardiovascular event, such as heart attack.

UnDiet Q&A: Where do I find potassium?

The recommended daily intake of potassium for all healthy adults is 4,700 mg. But most Americans only consume half the recommended amount. Bananas, beans, tofu, and potatoes are all rich sources of potassium. Many orange-colored fruits and vegetables are also good sources of potassium.

Food	Potassium Content
Edamame, ½ cup, cooked	970 mg
Sweet potato, 1 medium	541 mg
Potato	541 mg
Orange juice, 1 cup	538 mg
Apricots, 1 cup sliced	427 mg
Cantaloupe, 1 cup diced	427 mg
Banana, 1 medium	422 mg
Spinach, ½ cup, cooked	419 mg
Kidney beans, ½ cup	356 mg
Bok choy, ½ cup, cooked	315 mg
Pumpkin, ½ cup, mashed	281 mg
Chickpeas, ½ cup	238 mg
Orange, 1 medium	237 mg
Kiwi, 1 medium	237 mg

Table 2. Potassium-rich foods

Try baking, roasting, or steaming when cooking vegetables. Avoid boiling, as potassium leaches out into the water during cooking. Speak to your doctor before taking potassium supplements, especially if you have kidney-related health problems.

Don't Go To Extremes
Not All Processed Foods Are Bad For You

You've just read about some of the tricks manufacturers use in the production of processed foods to make them appear healthier than they are, and that processed foods are often loaded with sodium and chemicals. But the truth is, not all processed foods are bad for you. Just like your grandmother's canned peaches, a number of common processed foods can actually be good for you.

Olive oil, for example, is a processed food—the unprocessed version would be fresh, raw olives. Bread is processed by machines, and yet many versions found on store shelves have natural ingredients and are quite healthy. In fact, even if you make your own bread at home, you're still using processed products—flour itself is processed wheat.

Theoretically, it could be possible for all of us to mill our own flour or culture yogurt and cheese at home, but realistically that's just not going to happen! So, there's no need to go to extremes and avoid all processed foods.

UnDiet Q&A: 10 packaged foods that are good for you

1. Wine
2. Natural yogurt
3. Natural nut butter
4. Canned beans with no salt added
5. Frozen vegetables
6. Whole grain pasta and rice
7. Nuts
8. Dried fruits
9. Chocolate
10. Canned fish

Cut Out the Worst Offenders

Most people's biggest obstacle is overeating. What I mean by over-eating is not necessarily overeating during a meal. It's most likely eating when you don't need to eat. In other words, you may be snacking when you're not hungry. Do you snack while watching a movie in the theatre? Do you snack while taking a break at work? Do you snack while watching a sports game on TV?

It's so easy to over-snack. Back in your grandma's era, it was hard for people to overeat! If someone wanted to eat, they needed to go to market, bring home meat, veggies, and grains, and cook them. So much work for a 500-calorie meal. Now, you just need to open a bag of chips, and you can chow down 400 calories.

It is important to cut back on processed foods. After all, despite the fact that we have vast areas of agricultural land and access to fresh meat, dairy, and produce all year round, Americans seem to be addicted to processed food. A *New York Times* article reported that "Americans eat 31% more packaged food than fresh food."[6] The article also makes a good point about the different kinds of processed foods we eat, and why some of them are worse for us than others. Some Europeans, the article says, eat nearly as much processed food as we do. But they're eating bread from bakeries and cheeses from local shops, while we're eating "frozen toaster pastries and artificial nondairy creamer."

So, what are the worst offenders when it comes to processed foods we should avoid? Remember that *highly* processed foods (HPF) are the worst. The further removed any food is from its natural state, the more likely it is that it's had artificial ingredients added along the way, while fiber and vitamins may have been removed. So frozen cut vegetables are much less processed than, say, a frozen pizza, which is itself less processed than

Froot Loops. Here are some key things to avoid when choosing processed foods:

- **Colorings:** The Froot Loops mentioned above are a prime offender in this category, as are many other products aimed at kids. If you wouldn't find the color of a product in nature, you probably shouldn't eat it. The following is the ingredient list[7] on Kellogg's Froot Loops with colorings highlighted in bold:

  INGREDIENTS: SUGAR, WHOLE GRAIN CORN FLOUR, WHEAT FLOUR, WHOLE GRAIN OAT FLOUR, OAT FIBER, SOLUBLE CORN FIBER, PARTIALLY HYDROGENATED VEGETABLE OIL (ONE OR MORE OF: COCONUT, SOYBEAN AND/OR COTTONSEED OILS), SALT, SODIUM ASCORBATE AND ASCORBIC ACID (VITAMIN C), NIACINAMIDE, REDUCED IRON, NATURAL ORANGE, LEMON, CHERRY, RASPBERRY, BLUEBERRY, LIME AND OTHER NATURAL FLAVORS, **RED #40, BLUE #2, TURMERIC COLOR, YELLOW #6,** ZINC OXIDE, **ANNATTO COLOR, BLUE #1,** PYRIDOXINE HYDROCHLORIDE (VITAMIN B6), RIBOFLAVIN (VITAMIN B2), THIAMIN HYDROCHLORIDE (VITAMIN B1), VITAMIN A PALMITATE, BHT (PRESERVATIVE), FOLIC ACID, VITAMIN D, VITAMIN B12.

- **Preservatives:** How long can you keep fresh chicken breast in your fridge? I'd say at most three days. So how can some meat products, like wieners, last for weeks? Well, preservatives are added to make them last longer. The following is the ingredient list of Oscar Mayer's Classic Wieners.[8] All the sodium ingredients here are meant to extend shelf life.

  INGREDIENTS: MECHANICALLY SEPARATED TURKEY AND MECHANICALLY SEPARATED CHICKEN, PORK, WATER, CONTAINS LESS THAN 2% OF SALT, GROUND MUSTARD SEED, SODIUM LACTATE,

CORN SYRUP, DEXTROSE, SODIUM PHOSPHATES, SODIUM DIACETATE, SODIUM ASCORBATE, SODIUM NITRITE, FLAVOR.

- **Chemicals:** Mixes for baked products like cakes and muffins are the prime offenders here. When you bake from scratch, the list of ingredients is simple. But take a look at the ingredients list on a cake mix and you'll find that the ingredients sound like they belong in a lab, not a kitchen. These mixes don't really save much time anyway—you're better off to find a simple recipe that might take 10 extra minutes to make. For instance, take a look at the ingredient list[9] of Betty Crocker's SuperMoist Triple Chocolate Fudge. How many chemical-sounding ingredients can you find?

   INGREDIENTS: ENRICHED FLOUR BLEACHED (WHEAT FLOUR, NIACIN, IRON, THIAMIN MONONITRATE, RIBOFLAVIN, FOLIC ACID), SUGAR, COCOA PROCESSED WITH ALKALI (RED DITCHED AND DARK DITCHED), CORN SYRUP, SEMI-SWEET CHOCOLATE CHIPS (SUGAR, CHOCOLATE LIQUOR, COCOA BUTTER, SOY LECITHIN, ARTIFICIAL FLAVOR [VANILLIN]), LEAVENING (BAKING SODA, SODIUM ALUMINUM PHOSPHATE, MONOCALCIUM PHOSPHATE), PARTIALLY HYDROGENATED SOYBEAN AND/OR COTTONSEED OIL, MODIFIED CORN STARCH, CORN STARCH, CONTAINS 1% LESS OF: SALT, PROPYLENE GLYCOL MONO AND DIESTERS OF FATTY ACIDS, DISTILLED MONOGLYCERIDES, SODIUM STEAROYL LACTYLATE, DICALCIUM PHOSPHATE, XANTHAN GUM, CELLULOSE GUM, ARTIFICIAL FLAVOR.

- **Sodium:** We've already covered this common packaged food problem, but remember to try to avoid it whenever possible. In particular, avoid canned soup, instant noodles, and sodium-laden luncheon meat. A serving of frozen Digiorno Pepperoni Pizza has 940 mg of sodium. A serving of fat-free ham[10] has a whooping 820 mg of sodium. The same amount of roasted pork tenderloin has only 36 mg.

If you can cut down on HPF, you'll be taking a positive step to improve your diet. But don't feel guilty if you use frozen vegetables or canned fish—remember that these processed foods are actually good for you.

Go UnDiet Action #7: Un-shun all boxes.
You need to cut out the worst offenders and other "snack" foods. But don't feel like you have to avoid *all* processed foods. Some processed foods are actually good for you!

The 5-Second Scan: What to Look For
What's the 5-Second Scan?

The 5-second scan is a set of three quick tests you can use to evaluate the quality of a processed food within just 5 seconds of picking up the box. No matter how busy we are, most of us can spare at least 5 seconds to evaluate the products that we put in our shopping carts.

1. Watch Out for Colorful Characters

The sad truth is that many of the worst offenders for added sugar, sweeteners, and coloring are products marketed to kids. Cartoon characters on a box can be a quick clue that what's inside is more sugar than cereal. In fact, in a packaged food review I did for my website, I've reviewed more than 100 cereals. I found that the top 10 for highest sugar all had cartoon characters on the box. (Results of the Go UnDiet review: http://www.healthcastle.com/highsugarcereals) Some kids' cereals, including Apple Jacks, Froot Loops, Honey

Smacks, and Golden Crisp have sugar as the first ingredient! There are much healthier options in the cereal aisle. If your kids absolutely love one of these sugar-laden cereals, be sure to serve it only as a treat, or mix it with plain oat or bran cereal to minimize the amount of sugar and coloring your kids actually consume.

Go UnDiet Action #8: Un-cartoon.
Avoid products with cartoon characters on the box.

2. Fat-free Food is Not Real Food!

We've already talked about products that claim to be low-fat, and how manufacturers can trick you into thinking a product is healthier than it is. But when a product boasts that it's fat-free, I recommend you flat-out walk away. The simple truth is that fat-free food is not real food!

To replace fats in products that naturally contain fat, manu-facturers have to add thickeners or other artificial ingredients. The truth is that fat-free yogurt is just some milk ingredients with artificial thickeners added. And fat-free salad dress-ing, since it can't contain oil, is a Frankenstein's monster of artificial ingredients. Check out the ingredients[11] in Kraft's fat-free Italian salad dressing.

INGREDIENTS: WATER, VINEGAR, HIGH FRUCTOSE CORN SYRUP, CORN SYRUP, SALT, CONTAINS LESS THAN 2% OF PARMESAN CHEESE (PART-SKIM MILK, CHEESE CULTURE, SALT, ENZYMES), GARLIC, ONION JUICE, WHEY, PHOSPHORIC ACID, XANTHAN GUM, POTASSIUM SORBATE AND CALCIUM DISODIUM EDTA AS PRESERVATIVES, YEAST

EXTRACT, SPICE, RED BELL PEPPERS, LEMON JUICE CONCENTRATE, GARLIC, BUTTERMILK, CARAMEL COLOR, SODIUM PHOSPHATE, ENZYMES, OLEORESIN PAPRIKA.

That's a whole lot of "stuff" to drizzle on your salad, all for a savings of 40 calories per serving over the regular Classic Italian Vinaigrette.

 Go UnDiet Action #9: Un-fat-free.
Forget the fat-free claim. Fat-free products often bear little resemblance to real food, and are filled with additives.

3. Look at the Nutrition Facts AND the Ingredients List

Starting in the late '90s, we became obsessed with the Nutrition Facts panel on our foods. It's a helpful tool, but it doesn't tell you everything you need to know about the food you're buying. The other half of the equation is to look at the ingredients list.

A recent example of letting Nutrition Facts get in the way of sensible food judgment is a decision by New York City to ban homemade goods at school bake sales in favor of a list of approved items that, strangely, includes such products at Doritos and Pop-Tarts. The city's logic is that they can't check the calories and fat content of the homemade goods, so they don't know whether they meet the guidelines for food sold in schools, which include a maximum calorie count of 200 per serving.[12] But while certain kinds of Doritos and Pop-Tarts may have good numbers on their Nutrition Facts panels, they look a bit dodgy when you check out the ingredients list. Here are the ingredients[13] for Doritos Reduced Fat Cool Ranch chips, which, at 130 calories per single serving, is approved for sale in schools under New York's guidelines.

> **INGREDIENTS:** WHOLE CORN, VEGETABLE OIL (CONTAINS ONE OR MORE OF THE FOLLOWING: CORN, SOYBEAN AND/OR SUNFLOWER OIL), BUTTERMILK, SALT, CORN DEXTRIN, TOMATO POWDER, CORN STARCH, WHEY, CORN SYRUP SOLIDS, ONION POWDER, GARLIC POWDER, MONOSODIUM GLUTAMATE, CHEDDAR CHEESE (MILK, CHEESE CULTURES, SALT, ENZYMES), NONFAT MILK, SUGAR, DEXTROSE, MALIC ACID, SODIUM ACETATE, ARTIFICIAL COLOR (INCLUDING RED 40, BLUE 1, YELLOW 5), SODIUM CASEINATE, DISODIUM PHOSPHATE, SPICE, NATURAL AND ARTIFICIAL FLAVORS, DISODIUM INOSINATE, AND DISODIUM GUANYLATE.

Even at only 130 calories per serving, would you really rather have your kid eat that list of additives, sweeteners, and colorings than a slightly higher-calorie homemade cookie or brownie?

The Ingredients List: What to Look For

There are two key things to look at when you check a product's ingredient list. The first is how long the list is. In general, the more ingredients on the list, the more processed the food. However, this doesn't necessarily mean that products with the fewest ingredients are always the healthiest. It depends what the ingredients are. For example, corned beef has just five ingredients: beef, water, salt, sugar, and sodium nitrite. But that doesn't mean it's good for you! With added sugar, salt, and sodium, this is a processed food that is worth avoiding, even though it has a short ingredients list.

Act II Kettle Corn has only four ingredients: popping corn, palm oil, salt, and sucralose. But since palm oil is loaded with saturated fat, and sucralose is an artificial sweetener, this is another product with few ingredients that's worth avoiding. In fact, this product gives popcorn—a whole grain snack that is very healthy when air popped—a bad name, just by adding two ingredients.

We can also compare Haagen-Dazs Five milk chocolate ice cream, which prides itself on having only five ingredients (skim milk, cream, sugar, egg yolks, and cocoa processed with alkali[14]), with Horizon Organic chocolate ice cream, which has six ingredients (organic nonfat milk, organic cream, organic sugar, organic cocoa processed with alkali, organic guar gum, and organic carob bean gum[15]). The surprise is that the product with six ingredients actually has 100 fewer calories per cup, as well as less fat, fewer carbs, and less sugar. Five ingredients are not necessarily better than six. Just remember that in general, a shorter ingredients list is better than a long one.

The second thing to look for when you check the ingredients panel is whether or not you recognize most of the ingredients. A longer list may be okay on, for example, a can of vegetable soup that lists many vegetables as ingredients. But when the ingredients look like artificial sweeteners or sodium, or sound like components of your kid's next science experiment, this is a clue to put the product back on the shelf!

Go UnDiet Action #10: Un-panel.
Don't just look at the Nutrition Facts Panel. Also check the ingredients list before deciding to buy a product. Look for products that have the calorie and fat counts you're hoping for, without a ton of unrecognizable artificial ingredients.

Now that you know how to spot HPF, and understand why they're the weakest link, here are three foolproof ways to avoid them.

Three Foolproof Ways to Avoid the Weakest Link

Highly processed foods are always packaged and designed to be mass produced, and can stay on shelves for a long time. Here are three foolproof ways to avoid HPF when you shop.

1. **Don't buy your groceries at convenience stores or discount department stores.**

   Instead, shop at food markets. There are two ways to tell if the store you're in genuinely wants to sell you healthy food. First, when you walk into the store, do you see fresh produce, or packaged boxes? Food markets will always have fresh produce the moment you walk in. Second, check their flyers. On the front and back pages, do they feature fresh food, like produce and meat? Or do they feature boxed items? Again, food markets always feature fresh food.

2. **Does it look fresh?**

   Ask yourself this question: Does the food you're buying look fresh? You would never order a dish in a restaurant that was made a month ago, so why would you settle for that at home? HPF usually offer convenience—you can just open the box and eat the product with minimal preparation. So try to avoid HPF that are prepared in advance, like canned soup, canned pasta, frozen dinners, and frozen pizza. Once you are used to the idea of eating fresh foods, you will feel awkward eating a box of un-fresh HPF.

3. Can you make it at home?

Sofia Layarda, MPH, RD, my Assistant Editor at HealthCastle. com, uses the word "over-engineered" to describe HPF that are impossible to recreate at home. When you cook pork, is it pink like the ham slices you buy in shrink-wrapped plastic? Mine isn't. Can you make blue icing at home without adding food coloring? What about brown cola drinks? If you can't make it yourself, it's not natural.

Since I've called out over-snacking as the worst offending source of HPF, what should you snack on? Don't worry. I'm not saying we shouldn't snack. I just say that we shouldn't snack if we're not hungry. Certainly, if you need to snack, you can choose from the list of 30 healthy snacks under 200 calories, compiled in Appendix C by Beth Ehrensberger, MPH, RD, a contributing writer at HealthCastle.com.

5 Small Steps to UnDiet

Here's a review of the 5 UnDiet Actions you learned in this chapter. These small steps all take place at the grocery store, so here's what to think about the next time you head out to shop.

- ▶ **#6. Un-low.** Look for products that have a low-sodium claim, rather than focusing on low-sugar or low-fat.

- ▶ **#7. Un-shun boxes.** Cut out the worst offenders! For this week, try to leave one or two of your usual processed purchases on the shelf.

- ▶ **#8. Un-cartoon.** Avoid products with cartoon characters on the box. They're a sure sign that the product contains loads of sugar, and probably artificial coloring.

▶ **#9. Un-fat-free.** If it says fat-free, put it back on the shelf. Remember, fat-free food is not real food!

▶ **#10. Un-panel.** Check both the Nutrition Facts panel and the ingredients list. A shorter ingredients list is generally better than a long one, but also keep an eye out for unpronounceable mystery ingredients—which you should avoid.

CHAPTER 3

Re-learn Your Fats

You've probably been told that fat should make up about 30% of your total energy intake, and that you shouldn't get more than 10% of your energy from saturated fat. But you can forget about these numbers. They really don't mean anything to you in terms of planning what to get from your grocery store—and that's why I won't focus on them in this chapter.

Are Bad Fats Really That Bad?

You've heard the story about good fats versus bad fats. You may immediately identify trans fat and saturated fat as the bad guys. But are they really that bad? You've heard news of New York City banning the use of trans fat in restaurants. And you try to choose products that have a zero-trans-fat claim. But do you really know if a product is trans-fat free?

Trans Fat

Trans fat was "born" when food manufacturers started searching for an option to replace the bad saturated fat in their products. Food scientists quickly learned that by partially hydrogenating liquid oil, they could produce a stable, solid fat that was suitable for mass-scale food manufacturing. Trans fat is the by-product of this hydrogenation process. What these food scientists did not know, but later studies have shown, is that trans fat is actually as bad as, or even worse than, saturated fat. Studies have also shown that a diet high in trans fat may be linked to a greater risk of heart diseases, type 2 diabetes, and cancer.

Because of these findings, the U.S. government imposed a mandatory trans fat labeling ruling effective January 2006, making it a requirement to disclose trans fat information on food labels. New York City also has banned the use of trans fat in its restaurants since July 2008. Even with these measurements, however, trans fat is still lurking in our food system.

So, how much trans fat is too much? Well, in April 2004, the FDA Food Advisory Committee voted in favor of recommending that trans fatty acid intake be reduced to "less than 1% of energy." That's about 2 grams of trans fat per day for an average adult.

Don't be too excited, though, when you pick up a product that says "zero trans fat" or has 0 grams of trans fat on its Nutrition Facts label. Upon investigation, I've found numerous products with no trans fat listed on the label that still contain partially hydrogenated oil (a source of trans fat)—including chips, cookies, cereal, frozen pizza, salad dressing, and more. For example, Kraft Light Caesar salad dressing shows 0 grams of trans fat on its label. But if you look carefully at the ingredient list,[16] you will find partially hydrogenated oil.

INGREDIENTS: WATER, SOYBEAN OIL, VINEGAR, CORN SYRUP, PARMESAN AND ROMANO MADE FROM COW'S MILK CHEESES (PART-SKIM MILK CHEESE CULTURE, SALT, ENZYMES), SALT, SUGAR, EGG YOLKS, CONTAINS LESS THAN 2% OF GARLIC, MODIFIED FOOD STARCH, CITRIC ACID, XANTHAN GUM, LEMON JUICE CONCENTRATE, ANCHOVIES, DRIED CORN SYRUP, HYDROLYZED SOY PROTEIN, SPICE, POLYSORBATE 60, NATURAL FLAVOR, DEFATTED SOY FLOUR, VITAMIN E, DRIED GARLIC, **PARTIALLY HYDROGENATED COTTONSEED AND/OR SOYBEAN OIL,** WHEAT, TAMARIND, SOYBEANS, CARAMEL COLOR, MALTODEXTRIN. CONTAINS: MILK, EGG, ANCHOVY, SOY, COTTONSEED, WHEAT.

This happens because our food labeling law gives manufacturers a loophole of claiming 0 grams of trans fat if a product contains less than 0.5 grams per serving. You may not bother to take note of this, thinking 0.5 grams of trans fat in a serving of salad dressing isn't so bad. But the fact is, if most products you eat are taking advantage of this regulatory loophole, you may be eating more trans fat than you know.

 Go UnDiet Action #11: Un-miss partially hydrogenated oil.
You won't find partially hydrogenated oil in natural foods. They are only present in processed food. HPF like frozen pies and pastries, glazed doughnuts, and bottled salad dressing are the worst contenders for being sneaky in trans fat labeling.

Just when we think we know everything, there's always a twist. It turns out that not all trans fats are bad. One kind of trans fat may actually be good for you. Have you ever noticed that some milks and butters list trans fat on their Nutrition Facts labels? This is naturally occurring trans fat—conjugated linoleic acid (CLA) and vaccenic acid—which is found in beef, veal, lamb, and dairy products. These natural trans fats are not bad fat at all. Animal studies on the health implications of CLA, which contains one trans bond, are mostly positive. A scientific review found that CLA might have unique biological effects in decreasing body fat deposition, as well as a potential ability to prevent heart disease and cancer. The scientific committee does not support eating more meat to boost CLA intake,[17] but CLA is just another point to show not all animal fat is as harmful to your health as once thought.

Saturated Fat

We've all heard it—saturated fat in meat has been shown to raise total cholesterol and the bad LDL cholesterol. Early studies done in the '60s suggested alarming negative consequences of eating saturated fat,[18] which encouraged the public to label saturated fat as a "bad" fat.

What you may not know is that there are at least four types of saturated fats, but only three of them are bad! The three bad saturated fats—lauric acid, myristic acid, and palmitic acid—are mostly found in tropical plant oils. These solid, tropical plant oils are found in HPF as coconut oil or palm oil. Myristic acid is the worst in terms of cholesterol-raising effects.

The fourth saturated fat—stearic acid—is mostly found in meat and animal products, including dairy. It doesn't increase your cholesterol. In fact, it may do just the opposite. Some studies conducted in the '90s actually showed that stearic acid can lower total and LDL cholesterol,[19] maybe as much as monounsaturated fat (a predominant fat found in olive oil) in terms of cholesterol-lowering effect.[20] So, we don't really have to worry about stearic acid at all. It may not be good enough to be named a "good" fat, but it's definitely not as bad as we've been told. So I categorize it as a "neutral" fat—a fat we do not need to cut back on or increase.

In fact, we've often been told that meat contains bad fats, so we are fixated on the idea that we shouldn't eat too much of it. But the fact is, HPF may contain even more saturated fat (from tropical oils) than meat!

Food (100 g serving)	Total Fat (g)	Total Saturated Fat (g)
Pork		
Pork tenderloin	4.0	1.4
Ham (processed)	9.0	3.1
Chicken		
Chicken breast, skinless	3.6	1.0
Chicken breast, with skin	7.8	2.2
Chicken nuggets, frozen (processed)	19.82	4.0
Beef		
Ground beef, lean	11.7	4.6
Top sirloin beef	5.8	2.2
Beef pot pie, frozen entrée (processed)	11.4	4.1
Fish		
Fish, sole, baked	1.53	0.4
Battered fish sticks, frozen (~ 3½ sticks = 100 g) (processed)	13.25	2.8
Other		
Eggs (2 large = 100 g)	10.6	3.3
Chocolate chip cookies (processed, 100 g)	28.4	14.1

Table 3. Total fat and saturated fat content
Source: USDA National Nutrient Database for Standard Reference, Release 21

To put all of this information in perspective, Table 3 supports my recommendation of eating real, whole foods instead of HPF. Yes—steak and eggs have saturated fat, but cookies actually contain more saturated fat than ground beef! Processed frozen beef pot pie has twice as much fat as the sirloin steak of the same volume serving. Processed chicken nuggets have more than five times as much fat as chicken breast, and breaded fish sticks have eight times more fat than unbreaded! If you are a packaged food junkie, you are loading up on quite a bit of fat, as well as the bad kind of saturated fat found in the tropical plant oils used during processing. Switch your gear now! Instead of worrying about your meat and egg intake, focus on cutting back on HPF. We will discuss more on why you shouldn't worry too much about meat intake in Chapter 5.

 Go UnDiet Action #12: Un-HPF.
Yes, meat has saturated fat, but HPF actually has more! Choose one meal this weekend and involve your family in cooking all foods from scratch. Make it a family activity so you'll get extra pairs of helping hands.

Are Good Fats Really That Good?

The same story extends to the "good" fat category. You probably immediately identify fish and olive oil as the good fat sources. But the fact is, not all "good" fats are made equal. Some may not give you the positive health benefits you are hoping for!

Omega-3 Fat

We've heard a lot about the health benefits of omega-3 fat. It can lower total cholesterol, LDL cholesterol, and triglycerides, as well as boost the good HDL cholesterol. Recent studies have even found that eating fish may decrease the risk of developing breast cancer and colorectal cancer.[21] Other studies have also found that seniors who eat fish have lower cognitive decline![22]

Because of these findings, many of our foods are now fortified with omega-3. Between 2006 and 2008, the number of omega-3 fortified products alone increased by 68%, according to Mintel's Global New Products Database. Omega-3 is now added to various products—milk, juice, crackers, infant formula, breakfast cereals, and more. It seems that we are eating more omega-3 fortified foods, but are we eating the right kind of omega-3?

Omega-3: Plant vs. Marine

It turns out that not all omega-3 fats are created equal. DHA and EPA can only be found in marine sources, or extracted from micro-algae. The other, predominant, kind of omega-3—ALA—is found in plant sources such as nuts, seeds, soy, and cooking oil.

Most of the studies that have shown heart health benefits of omega-3 refer to the marine-based DHA and EPA. Numerous studies have confirmed that fish oil reduces triglyceride levels and boosts good HDL cholesterol levels. This prompted the American Heart Association to recommend using fish oil supplements as a measure to lower triglyceride levels in people with documented heart disease in 2002.

Few studies, however, have looked into the health effects of plant-based ALA. Studies have shown that ALA does get converted by our bodies into DHA and EPA, but the conversion rate is very low.[23] In addition, some studies question the safety of high-dose ALA, such as that found in flaxseed oils, as it's been shown that men who ingest high doses of ALA may have a higher risk of developing prostate cancer.[24] Although a systematic review[25] showed inconsistent findings, caution is warranted.

Go UnDiet Action #13: Un-plant omega-3.
Omega-3 fat from plants is not the same as omega-3 from marine sources. Only omega-3 from marine sources has been shown to offer heart-health benefits. Seafood is the main source of DHA/EPA. So pay attention to food products that claim to have omega-3. Do they actually contain DHA/EPA? Or just ALA?

So, are we eating enough marine-based DHA and EPA? How much should we eat? We are certainly not eating enough. According to the National Health and Nutrition Examination Survey, we are only eating one-fifth of the recommended 500 mg per day! Don't worry—it's really easy to reach that level. Just two servings of fatty fish per week will do the trick! (We will discuss fish in detail in Chapter 5 and fish oil/DHA supplements in Chapter 9.)

So, include at least 2 servings of seafood in your diet each week. For men, consume omega-3 from marine sources and stay away from concentrated plant-based ALA sources like flaxseed oil for now until more is known.

Omega-6 Fat

Early studies showed that omega-6 fat may decrease total and LDL cholesterol. However, later studies found that omega-6 may actually increase the risk of developing heart disease, cancer, and inflammation. In particular, a study found that more men died from stroke and heart attack with a diet higher in omega-6 fat.[26]

So, are we eating too much omega-6 fat? The American Dietetic Association reported that we certainly do get more omega-6 than we used to. An international organization went further to recommend reducing our intake of linoleic acid (a predominant type of omega-6).[27]

Not all scientific communities agreed with the recommendation of reducing omega-6 intake. But one point they all agree on is that our current intake of omega-6 is sufficient and there's no need to increase it. One theory is that too much omega-6 may throw off the balance of the omega-6/omega-3 ratio. Since both omega-3 and omega-6 lower LDL cholesterol, another position[28] suggested keeping the current level of omega-6 intake, but boosting omega-3 levels.

Because of the conflicting scientific results and recommendations, I'm categorizing omega-6 as a "neutral fat"—no need to cut back or increase.

> **Verdict: Use Less** omega-6-rich vegetable oils like safflower oil, low-oleic sunflower oil, grapeseed oil, and corn oil, as well as processed foods made with these oils.

Monounsaturated Fat (Omega-9)

Monounsaturated fat (MUFA), also known as omega-9, was made famous by olive oil in the Mediterranean diet. Found mostly in cooking oil, nuts, and avocados, MUFA was even touted as a fat buster in the 2008 book *Flat Belly Diet*. It may be a tall order to call MUFA a weight-loss miracle, but numerous studies have found health benefits in a high-MUFA diet. In particular, MUFA lowers total and LDL cholesterols when it replaces saturated fat, and it is found to be more effective in lowering cholesterol and triglyceride levels compared to a low-fat diet.[29] Independently, it can lower cholesterol levels, but it's not as effective as omega-3. Despite this,

I'm still categorizing MUFA as a "good" fat, as it is mainly found in plant-based foods.

> **Verdict: Eat More** nuts, seeds, and avocados, and stock your cupboard with vegetable oils like olive oil, high-oleic sunflower oil, and canola oil.

Summary

So, un-learn what you've been told about good fats and bad fats and re-learn your fats now. Not all saturated fats and trans fats are bad. Similarly, MUFA may not be as effective in lowering cholesterol as you may have thought. What all of this really means to you is that unless you are a chronic overeater, you do not really have to over-worry about which oil you use or about your meat and dairy intake. What you do need to pay attention to are those highly processed foods (HPF). As you saw in Table 3, many processed foods actually have more bad fats than your favorite steak.

> **The New Go UnDiet Fat Categories**
>
> **Good Fats:** Omega-3, MUFA (Omega-9)
>
> **Neutral Fats:** Omega-6, stearic acid
>
> **Bad Fats:** Trans fat but not naturally occurring trans fat (CLA), Saturated fat but not stearic acid

The Skinny on Cooking Oils

Cooking oil deserves a spot in this book because we use it every day! We use cooking oil as a heating medium at home, and we also use it as a seasoning agent. With a high smoke point and the ability to withstand high temperatures, some oils—like canola oil and peanut oil—are better cooking agents than others. But since this book's focus is on health (and not culinary skill), I will only discuss the nutritional aspects of cooking oil.

I am often asked to compare cooking oils. Every time I speak about nutrition in public, the question about cooking oil for home use is brought up. My answer is that all liquid oil is about the same. It's true! Unless you drink your cooking oil, or deep-fry every day, your choice of cooking oil doesn't make a huge difference. It's good that you pay attention to your cooking oil. But the fact is, the major source of oil in our diets isn't in home cooking—it's in packaged foods and fast-food meals!

Because we use cooking oil every day, the best kinds are those with high good fat content and low bad fat content. I've run an analysis on common cooking oils to find their good fat, neutral fat, and bad fat contents. Here's what I found.

Good cooking oils, containing 50% or more good fats:

Olive oil	Canola oil
Flaxseed oil	Sunflower oil
Avocado oil	Peanut oil

 Go UnDiet Action #14: Un-nitpick your cooking oil.
As the major source of oil doesn't come from home cooking, any cooking oil listed above is fine.

Bad cooking oils, containing 50% or more bad fats:

Coconut oil   Butter

Palm kernel oil   Palm oil

Take a look at Figure 1, which shows how much bad, good, and neutral fat is in each cooking oil.

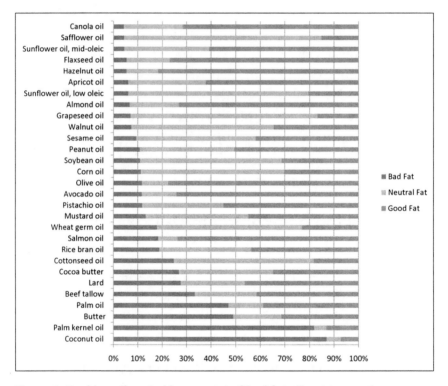

Figure 1. Cooking oil sorted by amount of bad fats (least to most)

Earlier, we talked about the bad kinds of saturated fat found in tropical oils, and this is where it all comes together. Coconut oil, for instance, contains 87% bad fat. Palm and palm kernel oil are not much better. You are probably thinking, "I never cook with palm oil." It's true—these oils are rarely used in regular cooking in North American homes. But they are indeed prevalent in our food system, especially in our HPF. For instance:

Orville Redenbacher Microwave Popcorn—Buttery Flavor

INGREDIENTS: POPPING CORN, **PALM OIL,** SALT, POTASSIUM CHLORIDE, NATURAL AND ARTIFICIAL BUTTER FLAVOR, BUTTER, COLOR.

Nutrition info: 190 calories with 5 grams of saturated fat per serving

Popcorn in its natural form is a healthy whole grain snack. The microwave version contains 5 grams of saturated fat, but the air-popped version of the same portion size contains merely 0.25 g of saturated fat. Let's take a look at another popular convenience food.

Nissin Instant Noodles—Chicken Flavor (1 bag)

INGREDIENTS IN NOODLES: WHEAT FLOUR, **PALM OIL,** SALT, POTASSIUM CARBONATE, SODIUM CARBONATE.

Nutrition info: 470 calories with 10 grams of saturated fat per serving

Egg noodles, vermicelli, or spaghetti would never contain that many calories or that much saturated fat. Spaghetti, for instance, contains no saturated fat at all.

These examples really show what processing does to the nutritional value of your food. In this case, instant noodles are pre-fried to cut down your cooking time. The more instant or convenient a packaged food is, the more processing it has gone through. Often, solid fat is added in the processing.

You may ask, "Isn't palm oil good?" Promoters of palm oil have told you so. They said that palm oil is different from palm kernel oil, and that it is extracted from the fruit of the plant, not the seeds. They said the saturated fat found in palm oil is not the same saturated fat found in palm kernel oil. But really, we should strive to lower the TOTAL saturated fat intake, instead of focusing on which fatty acid profile is more favorable.

 Go UnDiet Action #15: Un-palm.
Check the ingredient list and look for common solid fats in packaged foods: palm or palm kernel oil. The presence of this solid fat is an indication that the product is likely highly processed.

What about Coconut Oil?

Coconut is hot. From coconut milk, coconut yogurt, and coconut creamer to coconut water and coconut oil, coconut food products are definitely on their way to stardom. Some farmers are even using coconut feeds for their chickens.

But what's the real story on coconut oil? It certainly has a long-standing track record. For centuries, it has been used by people throughout the tropical world. Coconut oil is the oil extracted from the meat of a mature coconut. Because it is primarily made up of saturated fatty acids, coconut oil is very heat stable and has a high smoke point, which makes it useful in cooking and frying. It is also why coconut oil is comparatively stable and does not become rancid quickly. Unlike the hydrogenated coconut oil used in HPF, the virgin or "refined, bleached, and deodorized" (RBD) coconut oil that is sold on store shelves, such as Spectrum Organics, does not contain trans fats. As coconut oil contains high levels of medium-chained triglycerides (MCT, a type of saturated fat), coconut oil supporters claim that this exotic oil can boost your metabolism, help you lose weight, and fight infections. But you should know that the scientific evidence in support of such claims is very weak. The only substantiated health benefit of MCT, according to Dr. Roger Clemens, who is a professor at the USC School of Pharmacy and spokesperson for the Institute of Food Technologists (IFT), is for patients with disorders such as cystic fibrosis or gastrointestinal diseases. In terms of the other promises made by coconut oil supporters, Dr. Clemens says simply, "Coconut oil seems to be another craze with hijacked science."

What about Nut Butter?
Rich in fiber, phytonutrients, cholesterol-lowering plant sterols, good fats, and antioxidants such as Vitamin E and selenium, nuts are nutrition powerhouses. So what about nut butters? They can also be a great source of protein, but make sure you choose all-natural nut butter. All-natural nut butter usually doesn't have additives, and is an excellent choice to replace butter or margarine for your morning toast.

For example, here is a very simple food label[30] from an all-natural peanut butter with only two ingredients:

Smucker's Natural Creamy
Peanut Butter

INGREDIENTS: PEANUTS, SALT.

But, the list becomes long and complicated with processed peanut butter, which offers convenience by saving you time because it doesn't require stirring before spreading:

Jif Creamy Peanut Butter

INGREDIENTS: MADE FROM ROASTED PEANUTS AND SUGAR. CONTAINS 2% OR LESS OF: MOLASSES, FULLY HYDROGENATED VEGETABLE OILS (RAPESEED AND SOYBEAN), MONO AND DIGLYCERIDES, SALT.

Look at the extra ingredients and additives found in this peanut butter![31] Are you really in that much of a rush? How much time does it take you to stir a jar of natural peanut butter?

Don't be discouraged if you can't find all-natural nut butters in the usual peanut butter aisle. They may be shelved in the natural foods section. Try going beyond peanut butter to try other natural nut butters like almond, soy nut, pistachio, hazelnut, sunflower, or cashew butter.

5 Small Steps to UnDiet

This chapter's Go UnDiet Actions are all about changing your perception of oil and knowing what to look for when deciding whether to purchase foods that have claims related to oils.

▶ **#11. Un-miss partially hydrogenated oil.** Look at the ingredients lists on the convenience snacks, cookies, and frozen entrées in your home. Find those that contain partially hydrogenated oil and put them aside.

▶ **#12. Un-HPF.** Try sticking to food in its most natural form possible and cut down on processed foods. Instead of focusing on how much meat or how many eggs you've eaten this week, channel that energy to the highly processed packaged foods instead.

▶ **#13. Un-plant omega 3.** If you are advised by your doctor to take fish oil to lower cholesterol, make sure you purchase fish oil only. Do not waste money on plant-sourced ALA, which does not have the same benefits.

▶ **#14. Un-nitpick your cooking oil.** Stock good cooking oils at home. You don't have to get just one oil. Have one oil, like canola oil or peanut oil, for cooking, and another, like extra-virgin olive oil, for seasoning.

▶ **#15. Un-palm.** Remember, no solid fats are good. So beware of foods made with solid fats, such as palm kernel oil and coconut oil.

Don't Be Fooled by a High-Fiber Claim

These days, we are bombarded with messages telling us to eat more fiber. Why? Fiber not only promotes health, it also helps reduce the risk for some chronic diseases like constipation, hemorrhoids, and diverticulosis. Fiber is also linked to preventing some cancers, especially colon and breast cancers. In addition, fiber may help lower LDL cholesterol (the bad cholesterol) and total cholesterol, thereby reducing the risk of heart disease. Furthermore, fiber can help lower blood sugar, helping to better manage diabetes.

You're probably aware that you should be eating more fiber than you are, but you might not realize how little you're actually consuming. The recommended daily amount of fiber is 38 g per day for men and 25 g for women. But surveys show that we're actually only eating half that much.

This has created a market for food products that claim to have high fiber or added fiber, as well as an increased focus on whole grains. But what do those claims really mean? Let's take a look at how to decode the different fiber claims used on everyday products at the grocery store.

The Real Deal on "Whole Grain" Claims
What Exactly is Whole Grain?

A grain is considered whole when all three parts—bran, germ, and endosperm—are present. Whole grains are often an even better source of key nutrients, including antioxidants and phytonutrients, B vitamins, Vitamin E, magnesium, iron and fiber, than fruits and vegetables. Refined grains, on the other hand, usually only contain the endosperm of the grain, stripping away many beneficial nutrients, which are found mostly in the bran and germ.

When most people think about whole grains, they immediately think of whole wheat. But there are many other whole grains besides wheat.

wild rice	bulgur
brown rice	popcorn
whole wheat	amaranth
oatmeal	millet
whole oats	quinoa
barley	sorghum
whole rye	triticale

Table 4. Common whole grains

How Much Whole Grain Do We Need?

In North America, we began paying serious attention to whole grains in 2005, when the American Dietary Guidelines singled out whole grains for the first time, recommending that half our grain intake be made up of whole grains. You may be surprised to learn that means each of us should be eating three servings of whole grains every day. But a study done by the National Cancer Institute showed that the average person eats less than one serving of whole grains per day.[32]

Quite simply, we are just not eating enough whole grains.

Why does it matter? There are many reasons. Whole grains have been shown to reduce the risk of heart disease by decreasing cholesterol levels, blood pressure, and blood coagulation. Whole grains have also been found to reduce the risks of many types of cancer. They may also help regulate blood glucose in people living with diabetes. Other studies have also shown that people who consume more whole grains consistently weigh less than those who consume fewer whole grain products.

How Many Grains?

Average Adult Female: 6–8 servings (3–4 servings should be whole grains)

Average Adult Male: 7–10 servings (4–5 servings should be whole grains)

The Scoop on "Whole Grain" Products

Since that 2005 recommendation, companies have been introducing new whole grain products like crazy. Back in 2000, there were only 165 new whole grain products released, according to market research firm Mintel. But in 2009, there were more than 3,000 whole grain product launches. It seems that any product that is made with grains now has a "whole grain" or "multi-grain" version, including popular crackers, breads, chips, and breakfast cereals. And manufacturers want you to know that their products contain whole grains, so they've plastered various whole grain logos on their product boxes, including logos that say "Made with Whole Grains," "Good Source of Whole Grain," "Excellent Source of Whole Grain," or "100% Whole Grain." In some cases, products that haven't changed at all have added these logos and claims, so that consumers are more inclined to buy them. But what do all these claims really mean?

The truth is that there's very little regulation when it comes to using whole grain claims on product packaging. Any product that has some whole grains in its recipe probably has a whole grain claim or logo on the box. What you need to know is that just because a recipe contains some whole grains does not mean that is it made with 100% whole grains. Cheerios, for example, have a prominent whole grain checkmark logo on the front of the box. It's true that they do contain whole grain oats. But they also contain other starches, including wheat starch and modified corn starch!

> **INGREDIENTS:**[33] WHOLE GRAIN OATS (INCLUDES THE OAT BRAN), MODIFIED CORN STARCH, SUGAR, SALT, TRIPOTASSIUM PHOSPHATE, WHEAT STARCH, VITAMIN E (MIXED TOCOPHEROLS) ADDED TO PRESERVE FRESHNESS.

The only whole grain labels that have standards attached are those from the Whole Grains Council. These labels are shaped like postage stamps, and they say WholeGrainCouncil.org on the side.

Go UnDiet Action #16: Un-favor whole grain logos.
Don't be tricked: A whole grain logo or checkmark
on the front of a package does not mean a product contains
100% whole grains.

What About Whole Grain White Bread? Or Wheat Germ?

In case that's not confusing enough, it gets even more complicated.
Some white breads claim to contain the goodness of whole grains.
But white bread is made with refined white flour, not whole wheat,
so how can this be possible? Let's take a look at the ingredients[34]
in Wonder Bread's "Made with Whole Grain White Bread."

INGREDIENTS: ENRICHED WHEAT FLOUR [FLOUR, BARLEY MALT,
FERROUS SULFATE (IRON), B VITAMINS (NIACIN, THIAMINE
MONONITRATE (B1), RIBOFLAVIN (B2), FOLIC ACID)],WATER,
WHOLE WHEAT FLOUR, HIGH FRUCTOSE CORN SYRUP OR
SUGAR, YEAST, WHEAT GLUTEN, BROWN RICE FLOUR, SOY FIBER,
CALCIUM SULFATE. CONTAINS 2% OR LESS OF: SOYBEAN OIL,
SALT, VINEGAR, CORNSTARCH, WHEAT STARCH, SOY FLOUR,
HONEY, DOUGH CONDITIONERS (SODIUM STEAROYL LACTYLATE,
DATEM, MONO AND DIGLYCERIDES, ETHOXYLATED MONO AND
DIGLYCERIDES, DICALCIUM PHOSPHATE, CALCIUM DIOXIDE AND/OR
AZODICARBONAMIDE), YEAST NUTRIENTS (AMMONIUM SULFATE,
AMMONIUM CHLORIDE, MONOCALCIUM PHOSPHATE AND/OR
AMMONIUM PHOSPHATE), ENRICHMENT [VITAMIN E ACETATE,
FERROUS SULFATE (IRON), ZINC OXIDE, CALCIUM SULFATE, NIACIN,
VITAMIN D, PYRIDOXINE HYDROCHLORIDE (B6), FOLIC ACID,
THIAMINE MONONITRATE (B1) AND VITAMIN B-12], CALCIUM
PROPIONATE (TO RETAIN FRESHNESS), WHEY, SOY LECITHIN.

There are two important things to notice here. The first is that,
while this product does contain some whole wheat flour, it is in

position number three on the ingredients list. In fact, this product contains more water than whole wheat. According to the Whole Grain Council, "If there are two grain ingredients and only the second ingredient listed is a whole grain, the product may contain as little as 1% or as much as 49% whole grain (in other words, it could contain a little bit of whole grain, or nearly half)."[35]

Second, look at all the stuff that's been added to the first ingredient—enriched wheat flour. All of those additions, and many of the other nutrients found later on the list under "enrichment" are meant to simulate the nutritional benefits of a whole grain product. We'll talk a little later on about why this doesn't work as well as consuming real, whole grains, but for now just keep in mind that it's something to watch out for.

Leaving the questionable whole grain claims of white bread aside, what about other terms we see on product boxes that sound like they indicate the presence of healthy whole grains, like multi-grain, durum wheat, wheat germ, 100% wheat, stone ground, and so on? It's no wonder we're confused—check the sidebar on page 54 for guidance on some of the other grain terms you may have seen on product labels.

The simple way to tell if a product contains whole grains is to ignore the claims on the front package and check the ingredients list. If a whole grain is listed as the first ingredient, the product is a good source of whole grains.

Go UnDiet Action #17: Uncover whole.
Look for "whole." If the ingredient list uses the word "whole," the product actually contains whole grains.

Resource Alert: Use our Go UnDiet Review Tool to compare popular bread options. http://www.healthcastle.com/product-listing.shtml?catid=7

UnDiet Q&A: How to spot whole grains

As you've seen, the word "whole" in the ingredients list is a guarantee that the product contains whole grains. But what about other common wheat and grain terms—are they whole grains? Use this table to know for sure.

Words You May See On Packages	What They Mean
• whole grain [name of grain] • whole wheat • whole [other grain] • stoneground whole [grain] • brown rice • oats, oatmeal (including old-fashioned oatmeal, instant oatmeal) • wheatberries	YES—Contains all parts of the grain, so you're getting all the nutrients of the whole grain.
• wheat flour • semolina • durum wheat • organic flour • multigrain (may describe several whole grains or several refined grains, or a mix of both)	MAYBE—These words are accurate descriptions of the package contents, but because some parts of the grain MAY be missing, you are likely missing the benefits of whole grains.
• enriched flour • degerminated (on corn meal) • bran • wheat germ	NO—These words never describe whole grains.

Source: The Whole Grains Council. http://www.wholegrainscouncil.org/whole-grains-101/identifying-whole-grain-products

Don't Limit Yourself to Whole Grain Bread
Whole Grains are Not Just for Breakfast

When most people think about adding more whole grains to their diet, they tend to focus on breakfast foods, like whole wheat bread and whole grain cereal. But whole grains are not just for breakfast. They can make great lunches or excellent side dishes on the dinner table, and don't take any more work than the old starch standbys—potatoes, white rice, and pasta. You saw a list of some common whole grains at the beginning of this chapter; our writer Beth Ehrensberger has highlighted these five whole grains that are easy to be incorporated into your family's dinner.

Top 5 Natural Whole Grains for Lunch and Dinner

All of the five whole grains below can be used as substitutes for pasta or rice, and the preparation times and techniques are similar, so there's no reason not to try adding one of these whole grains to your dinner tonight!

Barley: Barley's chewy, mild flavor makes it a great substitute for pasta. To get started, simply cook barley in water (1 part grain to 2 parts water) until tender, then toss with your favorite pasta salad ingredients: beans, veggies, feta, olive oil, or whatever else you crave. In cooler weather, add a handful of barley to soup, chili, or stew to add filling texture. A half-cup serving of barley has 16 grams of fiber, while the same size serving of pasta contains only about 2.

Millet: Though millet isn't a grain that you'll commonly find on restaurant menus, there's good reason to feature it regularly in your kitchen—a powerful punch of protein is hidden behind its sweet, nutty flavor. Millet may be small, but it's mighty: It contains almost twice the amount of protein found in white rice. Use millet in the same way as you would rice. To prepare, just cook one part grain to two and a half parts water or chicken stock until tender. Toss in mushrooms and onions for a great pilaf or make a substantial hot breakfast by simmering in a mixture of half juice and half water, and mixing in nuts, milk, and dried fruit.

Bulgur: Bulgur is sold pre-cooked and dried, and it makes a good substitute for pasta. The great thing is there's no pot to watch—just pour boiling water over bulgur and let it sit covered for 20 minutes. Bulgur is the base of a classic favorite, tabouleh, which can be transformed into a quick one-handed lunch when loaded into a whole grain pita along with a bit of hummus. Try adding bulgur to sautéed fresh garden veggies like peas, onions, and zucchini with a little olive oil and garlic for a filling "bulgur primavera."

Quinoa: Since quinoa is actually a complete protein as well as a whole grain (it contains all nine essential amino acids) it's perfect for vegetarians and those looking to add more satiety—but no meat—to their plate. To prepare, just add one part quinoa to two parts water and use it as you would rice or pasta. Create a make-ahead meal that freezes well by mixing quinoa with corn, low-fat cheese, Italian spices, and marinara sauce, then stuff into green bell peppers and bake. For a super-powered breakfast, mix cooked quinoa with milk and top with bananas, walnuts, and dried cranberries.

Brown rice: Brown rice is the same grain as regular white rice—brown rice is just the whole grain version. (Regular white rice has the bran and germ layers removed.) Brown rice takes more water to cook than white rice—about 2 cups water to one cup rice—and also takes longer, about 45–55 minutes on the stove. You can make it in large batches and freeze the extras to reheat in the microwave at your next meal. Once you get used to brown rice, you may find that your family actually prefers its slightly nutty taste to plain white rice!

UnDiet Q&A: Tired of brown rice and whole wheat pasta?

Brown rice and whole wheat pasta are probably the most popular whole grain items on your dinner plate. If you are tired of eating them every night, but aren't ready to cook quinoa or millet yet, don't fuss—try Asian noodles first!

Chances are, you have eaten udon and soba at sushi restaurants, or vermicelli and rice noodles at Chinese restaurants. The good news is that whole grain versions are available! They don't often have flashy packaging with whole grain logos, and are often imported from Japan or Taiwan.

Soba
Soba's brownish noodles are made from buckwheat flour. They are available in a dried format in Asian grocery stores. Not all soba, however, is made from 100% buckwheat flour. Sometimes it includes refined flour, and sometimes whole wheat or spelt flour. So make sure to check the ingredient list and choose one that is mixed with whole grain flour, or made with 100% buckwheat.

Brown Rice Noodles
Rice noodles and vermicelli are popular in Asian cooking, so it's no surprise that brown rice versions are available. You don't usually find them on the menu in Chinese restaurants, but you can find the dried noodle packages in some Asian grocery stores. The ingredient list is usually simple: brown rice and water.

Whole Wheat Udon
The chewy udon you eat in sushi restaurants is made with refined wheat flour. But whole wheat or brown rice udon can be found in some Asian grocery stores, in either dried or frozen formats. Eden Foods even makes udon varieties made with kamut and spelt, too!

Don't forget that popcorn is also a whole grain, and it makes an excellent low-calorie snack at any time of day. Just be sure not to load it down with a ton of butter and salt!

 Go UnDiet Action #18: Unleash whole grains from breakfast.

Let whole grains make a grand entrance onto your dinner table, instead of limiting them to breakfast.

Added Fiber Does Not Equal Health Food

Food companies know that we are looking for more fiber and whole grains, but adding fiber to a food does not make it a health food.

Not All Fibers Are Created Equal

The positive impact of the 2005 Dietary Guidelines is that we are now paying more attention to fiber. We all know that fiber is good for us, and most of us even understand the importance of including more fiber in our diets. This, of course, has led food manufacturers to add fiber to many different products, hoping we will pick them up off the shelf because of that high-fiber claim. In fact, since fiber is now added to so many products, it can turn up where you'd least expect it—for example, in dairy products like yogurt and ice cream. Fruit juice and snack bars also often have added fiber. So are these products a good way to fill your daily fiber needs?

The short answer is no. The reason is because, as the heading for this section says, not all fibers are created equal. There are three types of fiber: soluble fiber, insoluble fiber, and isolated fiber.

Both soluble and insoluble fibers are undigested. They are therefore not absorbed into the bloodstream. Instead of being used for energy, fiber is excreted from our bodies.

Insoluble Fiber

Insoluble fiber helps move bulk through the intestines, and control and balance the pH (acidity) in the intestines. It promotes regular bowel movements and prevents constipation, removes toxic waste from the colon quickly, and helps prevent colon cancer by keeping an optimal pH in the intestines to prevent microbes from producing cancerous substances.

You can find insoluble fiber in green beans and dark green leafy vegetables, fruit skins and root vegetable skins, whole wheat products, wheat bran, corn bran, and seeds and nuts.

Soluble Fiber

Soluble fiber forms a gel when mixed with liquid. It binds with fatty acids, and prolongs the amount of time it takes for your stomach to empty, so that sugar in your food is released and absorbed more slowly. It lowers total cholesterol and LDL cholesterol (the bad cholesterol), thereby reducing the risk of heart disease, and can help regulate blood sugar for people with diabetes.

You can find soluble fiber in oats or oat bran, dried beans and peas, nuts, barley, flax seeds, fruits like oranges and apples, vegetables such as carrots, and psyllium husk.

Isolated Fiber

Isolated fiber—the fiber added to foods during processing—is not processed by the body in the same way as soluble and insoluble fiber. Studies have shown that some isolated fibers may be able to boost calcium absorption. However, no studies have shown that these isolated fibers offer benefits like their soluble and insoluble cousins. In other words, isolated fibers have not been shown to improve blood cholesterol levels or improve GI functions. It is thought the health-protective effect from foods containing fiber might be a synergy of the whole food, rather than the isolated fiber components.[36] So don't get too excited when you find products like ice cream bars with 6 g of fiber on the Nutrition Facts panel. Look at the ingredients list, and keep an eye out for these common isolated fiber ingredients.

Common Isolated Fiber Ingredients[37]

Inulin	Resistant maltodextrin	Pectin
Inulin from chicory root	Polydextrose	Gums
Maltodextrin	Indigestible dextrins	
Oat fiber	Resistant starch	

 Go UnDiet Action #19: Un-expect benefits from isolated fibers.
Skip the HPF that have fiber added. Isolated fiber does not work in the body the same way as natural fiber.

Natural Sources of Soluble and Insoluble Fiber
You've seen that the fiber found naturally in foods is processed differently from that added to foods. Not only do natural foods with natural fiber contain the beneficial types of fiber, they also contain all the nutrients and antioxidants associated with fiber. So how do you add more natural sources of fiber to your diet? It can be quite easy once you know all the places that natural fiber can be found. Take a look at Table 5, and try to replace some of the low-fiber or processed foods in your diet with natural foods that are naturally high in fiber instead.

enough fiber in your diet, even a small boost in fiber may shock your system enough to cause gas. Try adding fiber slowly to work up to the recommended levels of fiber intake without dealing with gas and bloating.

Sprouting, which is sometimes known as pre-germination, has a long history, but it's only recently that sprouted grain products have been making their way onto store shelves. Bread made from sprouted grains and sprouted brown rice are the most popular sprouted grain products, and also the easiest to find.

Health Benefits of Sprouted Grains

Sprouted grains, just like whole grains, contain all parts of the grain, so they offer all the same health benefits that whole grains do. Some sprouted grain products claim to have even better nutrition and increased protein content. So far, the studies seem to be backing these claims.

An early study found that sprouted cereal grains had an improvement in the amount of certain essential amino acids, total sugars, and B-group vitamins.[38] More recent studies have shown that sprouted brown rice has significantly higher levels of GABA, an important amino acid, than regular brown rice, as well as high dietary fiber and vitamin and mineral concentration in the bran and germ layers.[39,4]

Go UnDiet Action #20: Un-halt your grains; let them sprout.

Don't give up on the nutrition of whole grains because you don't like them. Try sprouted grains for a softer, easier-to-prepare version with improved nutrition.

5 Small Steps to UnDiet

This chapter's Go UnDiet Actions are all about getting more healthy fiber, including whole and sprouted grains, into your diet. So as you plan this week's meals and shopping list, keep all of these strategies in mind.

▶ **#16. Un-favor whole grain logos.** Don't be fooled! Remember that a whole grain claim on the front of the package does not mean a product is 100% whole grain.

▶ **#17. Uncover whole.** Look for the word "whole" in the ingredients list. Whole means it really is whole grains.

▶ **#18. Unleash whole grains from breakfast.** Don't limit your whole grains to breakfast. Try serving barley, millet, bulgur, quinoa, or brown rice at lunch or dinner.

▶ **#19. Un-expect benefits from isolated fiber.** Skip HPF with added fiber. Remember that "isolated" fiber is added fiber. Get your fiber from natural sources instead.

▶ **#20. Un-halt your grains; let them sprout.** Don't give up on whole grains just because you don't like whole wheat. Try sprouted grains for a softer texture with all the benefits of whole grains.

CHAPTER 5

You Don't Need to be Vegan to Eat Healthy

I often hear people say, "No meat for me tonight—I'm on a diet." But meat is not the diet villain it's made out to be. In fact, there's no reason you need to cut meat out of your diet to have a healthy eating plan and lifestyle, or to lose weight. Meat is often associated with high fat and calories, but the simple truth is that meat is not what's making us fat. In Chapter 3, we talked about HPF in Table 3 and how they often have more fat than meat. We'll talk more about that in this chapter, so you can see how meat can be part of a healthy, balanced diet that won't interfere with your weight goals.

Don't Be Afraid of Meat
How Much Fat and How Many Calories does Meat Really Have?

We tend to think of meat as being full of fat and calories. But the truth is, reasonable servings of most meats are not at all high in calories or fat. Take a look at Table 6 to see how some common cuts of meat really stack up.

Meat (3 oz. serving)	Calories	Fat (g)	Saturated Fat (g)
Chicken			
Chicken breast with skin	167	6.6	1.9
Chicken thigh with skin	210	13.7	3.7
Beef			
Top sirloin steak	207	12.1	4.8
Prime rib	340	28.7	11.9
Pork			
Pork tenderloin	125	3.4	1.2
Pork sirloin chop	181	8.6	3.1

Table 6. Calories and fat in common cuts of meat
Source: USDA Nutrient Database

This information is based on a three-ounce serving of meat. That's about the size of a deck of playing cards. You'll notice, of course, that the calories and fat vary quite a bit depending on the meat you choose—prime rib, for example, has more than twice the calories and fat of chicken breast or pork tenderloin. But none of these meat servings are going to blow your daily calorie and fat counts out of the water. Even if you double the serving size to six ounces, everything but the prime rib still falls under 425 calories and 30 grams of fat. So why do we have the impression that meat is so full of calories and fat? The problem is that since meat is often viewed as the main dish—the foundation upon which an entire meal is built—we do often eat more than one, or even two servings, in a meal. Some steakhouses offer twelve-ounce steaks! That's four servings of meat on your plate! Obviously, portion size makes a huge difference here. But if you stick to a reasonable portion, meat can be a healthy part of your meals.

How Does Meat Stack Up Against HPF?

If meat's not the diet villain, what is? It's HPF—highly processed foods. All those snacks and drinks are the real culprits for our obesity epidemic. Take a look at Table 7. You'll see that most of these common snack items have as much (or more!) fat and calories as the cuts of meat shown above—but these snack foods offer no nutritional benefits, and are sometimes packed with ridiculous amounts of sugar, too.

Snack	Serving Size	Calories (kcal)	Fat (g)	Sugar (g)
Kit Kat	1 package	210	11	22
Coca-Cola cola drink	1 bottle	233	0	65
M&M's milk chocolate	1 bag	240	10	31
Snickers	1 package	280	14	30
Lay's potato chips	2 oz.	300	20	0
Nissin Cup Noodles	1 cup	300	13	2
Cheetos	2 oz.	320	20	2
Arizona Kiwi Strawberry drink	1 large can	345	0	81
Digiorno frozen pepperoni pizza	1 slice	380	17	7
McDonald's fries	large	500	25	0

Table 7. Calories, fat, and sugar in common snack foods and drinks

 Go UnDiet Action #21: Be unafraid of meat.
I'm not trying to convince you to eat more meat. I just want you to understand that meat is not the cause of our obesity problem. Pay attention to what you snack on and what you drink—that's where most empty calories come from.

So exactly how much meat?

Your meat intake depends on your calorie requirement. Check Appendix B for details. If you haven't determined your calorie needs yet, do so with our free Calorie Calculator http://www. healthcastle.com/calorie-requirement-calculator.shtml

---

How Much Meat?

Average Adult Female: 5–6.5 oz.

Average Adult Male: 6–7 oz.

What Do All the New Packaging Terms Mean?

Ever wonder what the difference is between grass-fed beef and organic beef—or why it matters? With many people wanting to buy meat that has not been treated with antibiotics or hormones, and wanting to know that the meat they're eating comes from animals who were raised in a humane way, a whole new set of terms have cropped up in meat labeling. Take a look at the sidebar for a quick guide to the new terminology you may find on meat packaging in the grocery store.

UnDiet Q&A: What do these meat terms mean?

Grass-fed beef: The cows are fed a diet of grass and forage instead of grain feed, with the exception of milk consumed before they are weaned.[41] Grass-fed beef is generally reported as lower in fat overall, and has higher levels of omega-3, CLA, Vitamin A, Vitamin E, and antioxidants, as well as lower levels of cholesterol.[42]

Certified organic beef: Cattle must be fed 100% organic feed, but may be given certain vitamin and mineral supplements. Animals are given no antibiotics or growth hormones, and must have access to pasture.[43]

Free-range chicken or turkey: The birds should have outdoor access. However, no standards are defined for stocking density, the frequency or duration of how much outdoor access must be provided, or the quality of the land the birds have access to.[44]

Free-run or cage-free chicken: Birds are not kept in cages, but they usually don't have access to the outdoors.

Certified humane: The animals must be kept in conditions that allow for exercise and freedom of movement: crates, cages, and tethers are prohibited. Outdoor access is not required for poultry or pigs, but is required for other animals, and stocking densities are specified to prevent overcrowding. Animals are not given hormones or non-therapeutic antibiotics, and must be provided with bedding materials.

Natural or naturally raised: Unfortunately, these claims are not regulated.

Hormone-free or no hormones added: You may see this label on beef or milk products, indicating that the cows are not injected with the growth hormones rBGH or rBST. Many developed countries, including Canada, Japan, Australia, and the European Union, have banned the use of rBGH. The problem with growth hormone is that it can cause mastitis—an infection in breast glands that may result in pus and blood in milk. To prevent this, antibiotics are often used in cows injected with rBGH. Again, the EU and Canada have also banned the use of antibiotics, but it's legal in the United States.

The problem, of course, is that these labels can significantly increase the price of meat products. I always buy free-range chicken, because for me, it's worth the extra cost—both because I know that the animals were treated better and because the chicken just tastes better. Take a look at the price differences in Table 8 and use it and the information in the sidebar to make your decisions about what kinds of meat to buy.

Meat	Price
Beef	
Ground beef, organic and grass-fed	$ 6.99/lb
Ground beef, antibiotics-free	$ 5.99/lb
Ground beef	$ 3.99/lb
Top sirloin, antibiotics-free	$ 6.99/lb
Top sirloin	$ 4.99/lb
Chicken	
Chicken breast, organic	$ 10.99/lb
Chicken breast, antibiotics-free	$ 4.29/lb
Chicken breast	$ 3.49/lb
Pork	
Center-cut pork loin chop, antibiotics-free	$ 6.99/lb
Center-cut pork loin chop	$ 4.99/lb
Eggs	
Brown eggs, organic, free-roaming	$ 3.99/dozen
Brown eggs, free-roaming	$ 2.89/dozen
Brown eggs	$ 2.19/dozen

Table 8. Cost differences for meat. Prices obtained on FreshDirect.com on Jun 17, 2010

 Go UnDiet Action #22: Un-medicate your meat.
Choose meat that's raised as naturally as possible. We always say, "You are what you eat." The same applies to animals. If their diet is good, and they lead a healthy life, the products they produce will be good too.

Excellent Eggs
Different Kinds of Eggs

Do you prefer brown eggs over white eggs? What about a dark yellow yolk over a pale yellow yolk? Did you know that these differences in color actually have nothing to do with the quality, flavor, freshness, or nutritional value of the eggs? Egg yolk color is determined by the type of feed a hen eats. A wheat-based diet will produce a pale yellow yolk, while a corn- or alfalfa-based diet yields a darker yellow yolk. In terms of shell color, it simply depends on the breed of hen laying the eggs. That said, there are a lot of different kinds of eggs on grocery store shelves. Let's take a look at the different kinds of eggs, and whether they're worth the extra money stores sometimes charge.

Omega-3 enhanced eggs are from hens fed a diet of flax seed or fish oils. Omega-3 enhanced eggs contain more omega-3 fatty acids and Vitamin E than regular eggs. An independent test conducted by the Canadian TV show Marketplace found that omega-3 enhanced eggs contain approximately seven times more omega-3 fatty acids than regular white eggs.

Organic eggs are produced by hens fed certified organic grains without most conventional pesticides and fertilizers. Growth hormones and antibiotics are also prohibited. Organic eggs have the same nutritional content, fat, and cholesterol as regular eggs.

Free-run or cage-free eggs are produced by hens that are able to move about the floor of the barn and have access to nesting boxes and perches. The nutrient content of these eggs is the same as that of regular eggs.

Free-range eggs are produced in a similar environment as cage-free eggs, but hens have access to outdoor runs as well. The nutrient content of these eggs is the same as that of regular eggs.

Processed eggs, such as liquid egg whites or dried egg whites, are shell eggs broken by special machines, then pasteurized before being further processed and packaged in liquid, frozen, or dried form. Processed egg products may also contain preservatives and flavor or color additives.

According to the Egg Nutrition Center, the nutritional value of an egg is affected *only* by the feed. In other words, specialty eggs such as organic eggs or cage-free eggs provide the same nutritional value as the regular varieties if their feeds are the same. The only specialty eggs with enhanced nutrition are omega-3 enhanced eggs.

An Egg is a Nutrition Powerhouse

Eggs are rich in protein, folate, Vitamin B12, and Vitamin D. They are also a good source of lutein, a type of antioxidant. Plus, just one egg can provide half your daily requirement of choline, an essential nutrient responsible for mental health and brain function. That's a lot of nutritional value crammed into one small package!

What About Cholesterol?

The cholesterol content of eggs has been a hot topic for more than 10 years. But there is no reason to fear eating eggs. It's true that eggs are high in cholesterol. However, there is no evidence that they are fattening, or that they will make you gain weight. And, despite its scary name, you shouldn't assume that cholesterol in foods is closely related to cholesterol in your blood. In fact, dietary cholesterol (the cholesterol you consume by eating foods like eggs) has less impact on your blood cholesterol than trans fat and saturated fat, which are mainly found in HPF.

That's why the American Heart Association does not mention limiting egg consumption as a way to help prevent heart disease.

There is just no evidence that eating an egg a day will increase your risk for heart disease, so it's fine to include eggs in your diet if you're not already facing heart disease risk.

If your cholesterol is high—especially your LDL (bad) cholesterol or triglycerides—the National Cholesterol Education Program recommends you eat no more than two egg yolks per day, but allows for unlimited egg whites. If you are at risk for heart disease, rather than worrying about eggs, you should focus on cutting down on trans fat and saturated fat, both of which are highly prevalent in HPF.

 Go UnDiet Action #23: Un-crate eggs.
While they are high in dietary cholesterol, eggs don't have a strong impact on blood cholesterol, and will not cause you to gain weight. The nutritional benefits make eggs a great, healthy choice.

Health Benefits of Seafood
Seafood's Unique Health Benefits
Many seafood options contain much lower calories, fat, and saturated fat than many meat products. Take a look at Table 9 to see how seafood stacks up against popular meat options.

Food (3 oz. serving)	Calories (kcal)	Fat (g)	Saturated Fat (g)
Meat			
Top sirloin steak, trimmed to 0" fat	180	8.2	3.2
Pork loin chop	141	3.6	1.3
Chicken breast with skin	167	6.6	1.9

Seafood			
Cod	89	0.7	0.1
Tuna, light, canned in water	99	0.7	0.2
Sole	99	1.3	0.3
Shrimp	84	0.9	0.3
Crab, blue	87	1.5	0.2
Scallop	95	1.2	0.1

Table 9. Calories, fat, and saturated fat in seafood and meat

As you can see, seafood's calories and fat numbers are impressive. But what actually makes seafood such a valuable addition to the diet is that it's one of very few foods that provide DHA and EPA—two essential fatty acids that have been shown to have a host of health benefits, from enhancing cognitive development in infants to lowering the risk of heart attack and death. Two servings of fatty fish per week can generally meet the daily recommended intake levels of DHA and EPA.

Seafood is also rich in selenium, a powerful antioxidant that protects against free radicals, helps regulate thyroid function, and boosts immunity. Selenium may even help reduce the risk of certain kinds of cancers, especially prostate cancer. An epidemiological study revealed that men with high blood levels of selenium were about half as likely to develop advanced prostate cancer as men with lower blood selenium.[45]

What About Mercury?

Thanks to all these health benefits, for a while, it looked like seafood was set to become the next big super food. Then, in March 2004, the Food and Drug Administration and Environmental Protection

Agency issued an advisory that stirred up concerns about mercury levels in fish. The warning was targeted at pregnant women and children under 12, and basically said that women who are pregnant or may become pregnant, nursing mothers, and young children should avoid certain types of fish (shark, swordfish, king mackerel, and tilefish), eat no more than one serving of albacore tuna per week, and focus on eating fish and shellfish that are lower in mercury.

But once the idea of mercury became associated with seafood, it scared off many people—not just pregnant women. And it scared them away from a much broader range of seafood than the ones that were part of the warning. As a result, many people are missing out on the excellent nutritional benefits of seafood because they're afraid of consuming mercury. This is really a shame, because the truth is that not all seafood contains mercury. In fact, in some seafood species, the level of mercury is so low as to be undetectable.

Species	Average Mercury Concentration (ppm)
Low Mercury (Enjoy a variety)	
Clam	Not detectable
Ocean perch	Not detectable
Salmon (canned)	Not detectable
Shrimp	Not detectable
Whiting	Not detectable
Tilapia	0.01
Oyster	0.013
Hake	0.014
Salmon (fresh/frozen)	0.014
Sardine	0.016
Haddock (Atlantic)	0.031
Crawfish	0.033

Pollock	0.041
Anchovies	0.043
Herring	0.044
Flatfish (includes flounder, plaice, sole)	0.045
Mullet	0.046
Catfish	0.049
Atlantic mackerel (N. Atlantic)	0.05
Scallop	0.05
Butterfish	0.058
Crab (includes blue, king, snow)	0.06
American shad	0.065
Whitefish	0.069
Squid	0.07
Croaker (Atlantic)	0.072
Trout (freshwater)	0.072
Chub mackerel (Pacific)	0.088
Lobster (spiny)	0.09
Cod	0.095
Jacksmelt	0.108
Tuna (canned, light)	0.118

Moderate Mercury (6 servings or less a month)

Sheepshead	0.128
Skate	0.137
Carp	0.14
Perch (freshwater)	0.14
Tilefish (Atlantic)	0.144
Lobster (species unknown)	0.169
Monkfish	0.18
Spanish mackerel (S. Atlantic)	0.182
Snapper	0.189

Buffalofish	0.19
Skipjack tuna (fresh/frozen)	0.205
Bass (includes sea bass, saltwater, black, striped, rockfish)	0.219
Sablefish	0.22
Halibut	0.252
Weakfish (sea trout)	0.256
Scorpionfish	0.286
White Croaker (Pacific)	0.287
Lobster (Northern/American)	0.31
High Mercury (3 servings or less a month)	
Yellowfin tuna (fresh/frozen)	0.325
Bluefish	0.337
Albacore tuna (canned)	0.353
Albacore tuna (fresh/frozen)	0.357
Tuna (fresh/frozen, all)	0.383
Chilean bass	0.386
Tuna (fresh/frozen, species unknown)	0.414
Highest Mercury (Avoid)	
Spanish mackerel (Gulf of Mexico)	0.454
Grouper (all species)	0.465
Marlin	0.485
Orange roughy	0.554
Bigeye tuna (fresh/frozen)	0.639
King mackerel	0.73
Swordfish	0.976
Shark	0.988
Tilefish (Gulf of Mexico)	1.45

Table 10. Amount of mercury in various types of seafood
Sources: U.S. Food and Drug Administration;[46] Natural Resources Defense Council and Natural Resources Defense Council[47]

As you can see in Table 10, many seafood choices, like clams, salmon, shrimp, tilapia, pollock, sardine, and catfish, have low or non-detectable levels of mercury. The recommendation on frequency of eating is really for pregnant women. Men, women who are not pregnant, and teenagers do not need to worry so much

UnDiet Q&A: Which seafood is sustainable?

These days, many people are just as concerned about sustainable fishing practices as they are about the nutritional value of the seafood they consume. Both the Environmental Defense Fund and the Monterey Bay Aquarium have ranked seafood sustainability in terms of fish population and fishing and farming practices. They both recommend the following seafood options as best eco-choices:

- Dungeness crab

- Mussels

- Farmed oysters

- Wild sablefish/black cod from Alaska and British Columbia

- Wild salmon from Alaska

- Sardines

- Pink shrimp from Oregon

- Farmed rainbow trout

- Albacore tuna from the U.S. and Canada

You can find the whole Environmental Defense Fund list at http://www.edf.org/page.cfm?tagID=1521 and the Monterey Bay Aquarium list at http://www.montereybayaquarium.org/cr/SeafoodWatch/web/sfw_factsheet.aspx.

about mercury in seafood, though of course it makes sense to choose lower-mercury species if you eat seafood often. Choose a variety of different kinds of seafood to get the maximum amount of nutritional benefits while minimizing your mercury exposure.

 Go UnDiet Action #24: Unveil fish.
Choose a variety of low-mercury fish as often as you wish. Pregnant or lactating women and kids under 12 should avoid high-mercury fish, but it's safe to eat up to four servings of low-mercury fish per week.[48] For everyone else, there's not as much concern about mercury, but it's a good idea to choose lower-mercury seafood anyway.

Processed Meat Landmines
What is Processed Meat? And is it Really That Bad?

Meats that are salted, cured, smoked, or preserved with nitrate are considered processed meats. This includes bacon, sausage, ham, hot dogs, salami, luncheon meat, and other cured meats. They are usually high in fats and salt, which means they are not heart-friendly. A slice of regular ham, for instance, contains two times more fat and 25 times more salt than an equivalent portion of pork tenderloin. Most processed meats contain nitrites and nitrates as preservatives, as well as coloring and flavoring additives. As you can see in Table 11, compared to their fresh, whole-cut meat counterparts, processed meats are typically higher in sodium, calories, and fats.

What's worse, processed meats have been linked to specific health problems, including cancer and food-borne illnesses like listeriosis.

Processed Meat (3-oz. serving)	Calories	Total Fat (g)	Sodium (mg)
Bacon, Canadian back	122	5.3	1,002
Bacon, center cut	354	28.4	1,914
Bacon, turkey	213	15.2	1,094
Beef, roast, cold cuts	138	3.5	32
Beef, slow roasted, 95% fat free (Oscar Mayer's)	100	4.2	867
Beerwurst pork, beer salami	202	16	1,055
Beerwurst, beer salami, pork & beef	236	19.1	623
Bologna, beef	267	24	919
Bologna, turkey	178	13.7	1,065
Chicken breast, oven roasted, 97% fat free (Oscar Mayer's)	90	2.2	1,059
Chicken breast, oven roasted (Oscar Mayer's)	92	2.6	1,060
Chicken breast, rotisserie (Oscar Mayer's)	83	1.7	800
Chorizo, pork & beef	387	32.6	1,050
Chorizo, traditional pork	231	18.2	826
Corned beef, saval, brisket	106	3	759
Ham, black forest	106	3.8	440
Ham, extra lean, 5% fat	94	2.5	941
Ham, honey	137	6.8	714
Ham, rosemary (principe)	182	3	1,200
Kielbasa, turkey and beef	192	15	1,021
Pepperoni	396	34.3	1,521
Prosciutto (German deli)	170	10.2	1,701
Salami, cold cuts, hard (Oscar Mayer's)	315	25.2	1,607
Salami, hard	273	18.2	1,519

Sausage, pork	259	22.5	541
Sausage, summer, beef	284	23.9	955
Sausage, summer, beef & pork	308	25.9	1,106
Summer sausage, beef (Oscar Mayer's)	273	21.3	1,215
Tuna, canned in water	109	2.6	321
Tuna, light, canned in water	99	0.7	287
Turkey breast meat	88	1.4	863
Turkey breast, smoked (Oscar Mayer's)	90	1.5	940
Weiner with natural casing	213	16.7	775

Table 11. Calories, fat, and sodium in processed meats
Source: Calorieking.com

Processed Meat and Cancer

A 2007 report[49] from the American Institute for Cancer Research and World Cancer Research Fund found a direct link between eating processed meat and developing certain kinds of cancer, including colorectal and lung cancers. The study concluded that eating a 50-gram serving of processed meat every day increases the risk of colorectal cancer by 21 percent. A 50-gram serving is approximately the same size as a hot dog, a product that many children eat on a regular basis! Researchers have not yet been able to pinpoint which ingredients in processed meats are responsible for the increased risk of cancer, but heme iron, nitrates, and nitrites have been brought up as possibilities and are being looked at.[50]

Processed Meat and Food Borne Illness

Listeria can be present in processed meats that do not seem spoiled in any way. Pregnant women, newborns, the elderly, and those with weakened immune systems are most susceptible to listeria.

Don't think food poisoning is all that big a deal? A 2008 listeria outbreak in Canada claimed the lives of 22 individuals, and there have been several recalls of processed meats due to listeria concerns since.

 Go UnDiet Action #25: Undo your relationship with processed meat.

Due to the increased risk of cancer (especially colorectal cancer), and of contracting listeria, children, the elderly, pregnant women, and people with weakened immune systems should not eat processed meat. Even if you do not fall into one of these categories, you should avoid processed meats if you can.

5 Small Steps to UnDiet

This chapter's Go UnDiet Actions invite you to get reacquainted with meat, eggs, and seafood, which can all be part of a healthy, weight-friendly diet.

- ▶ **#21. Be unafraid of meat.** It's not as high in fat or calories as many junk foods that get much less negative attention. Stick to healthy portion sizes and enjoy your meat!

- ▶ **#22. Un-medicate your meat.** Choose meat from animals that are raised as naturally as possible, and avoid growth hormones in particular.

- ▶ **#23. Un-crate eggs.** They've developed a bad reputation for being high in cholesterol, but eggs don't increase blood cholesterol or lead to weight gain, and they offer a ton of nutritional benefits.

- ▶ **#24. Unveil fish.** Not all fish is high in mercury. With its unique nutritional benefits, low-mercury seafood is an excellent addition to any dinner table.

- ▶ **#25. Undo your relationship with processed meat.** From cancer risk to food safety issues—never mind loads of sodium and food additives—processed meats should simply be avoided.

CHAPTER 6

Study Your Drinks

Every system in your body depends on water. Water flushes toxins from your body, carries nutrients to your organs, and provides a moist environment for your ear, nose, and throat tissues. How much water you need really depends on your activity levels, environment, and general health status, but the general consensus is that we need at least six cups of water a day. The Institute of Medicine actually recommends much more than that—suggesting 9 cups of fluids a day for women and 13 for men. But the truth is, hardly anyone actually drinks six or more cups of plain, unflavored, natural, zero-calorie water. So what are we really drinking—and how do the drinks we consume impact our overall health and weight?

Thirst-Quenchers or Weight-Gainers?
What Happened to Water?

Our beverage consumption patterns have shifted markedly during the 20th century, and they continue to evolve. In his study,[51] Dr. Barry Popkin found an increase in the consumption of sugar-sweetened drinks. Findings from the American Heart Association back this up as well. The AHA found that over the past 30 years, our total calorie intake has increased about 150–300 calories per day—and half of that increase comes from liquid calories, primarily in the form of sweetened drinks.[52] In fact, across all age groups, from toddlers to senior citizens, we now drink more calorie-containing drinks than we drink water. In particular, adults aged 19–39 drink an average of 533 calories every day![53] That's equal to a whole extra meal, and sugar-sweetened drinks are the main contributor to that stack of extra calories.

So, what exactly is considered a sugar-sweetened drink? I'm sure you know that soda is sweetened, but we drink a lot of sweetened beverages that fall outside the soda category.

Sugar-sweetened Drink (per 8 oz.)	Calories
Slurpee, 7-11, Coca-Cola Classic	65
Iced Tea, Arizona—Lemon	90
Sunny D Tangy Original	90
Coca-Cola—Regular	93
SoBe Energize Mango Melon	120
Arizona Kiwi Strawberry	120
Rockstar Energy Drink	140
White Chocolate Crème Frappuccino Blended Beverage, Starbucks	240
Strawberry Milkshake, McDonald's	280
Milkshake, Cold Stone's PB&C	670

Table 12. Calories in sugar-sweetened drinks

The worst part is, not only are these sweetened drinks high in calories, but those calories don't give you a feeling of being full.

That means that although you consume extra calories through your drinks, you don't end up eating any less food—so your total calorie intake just keeps creeping up each time you drink a sweetened beverage.

So, think about why you're consuming that beverage—is it really because you're thirsty? If so, stick to drinks that actually rehydrate your body without filling you up with sugar. Calorie-free tap water is a good choice, but tonic water with 125 calories may not be as good. A cup of green tea is a good choice, but a bottle of iced green tea with 200 calories may not be as good.

Go UnDiet Action #26: Un-drink your calories.
Drinks are meant to replenish your body's fluids— so good drink choices are those that do just that, without a ton of calories.

UnDiet Q&A: Which tea is good for you?

By now, just about everyone has heard that tea is a healthy drink choice because it contains high levels of antioxidant polyphenols. Indeed, tea ranks higher than some fruits and vegetables on the antioxidant scale. In fact, we've put green tea on our Top 60 Super Food list in Appendix D.

But, we tend to call a lot of things "tea" that aren't really tea—and don't have the health benefits of real tea. Only tea that is made from the leaves of the warm-weather evergreen Camellia plant is true tea, with all the antioxidant benefits you expect to find in tea. So the key question is, which teas are made from the Camellia plant? It's really very simple. Black tea, green tea, white tea, and oolong tea are all made from the Camellia plant, so they are all true teas that contain health-promoting polyphenols.

Herbal teas and red or rooibos tea, on the other hand, are not true teas. Technically, these are tisanes, meaning they are infusions made with herbs, flowers, roots, spices, or other parts of various plants. Therefore, herbal and rooibos teas, while they are fine if you're simply looking for a calorie-free warm beverage, do not offer the health benefits associated with true tea.

And what about iced tea? Many people think that since tea offers so many health benefits, iced tea must be a healthy drink option for the summer months. This may be true if you make your own iced tea using real black, green, white, or oolong tea. But all those people who say, "I don't drink soda; I drink iced tea" might be shocked to learn that bottled iced tea can actually be even worse than soda. If you pick up a bottle of iced tea and compare its ingredients to a can of soda, you can see the similarities quite clearly. Take a look at the ingredient list[54] for Lipton's Iced Tea with Lemon.

> **INGREDIENTS:** WATER, HIGH FRUCTOSE CORN SYRUP, TEA, CITRIC ACID, SODIUM HEXAMETAPHOSPHATE (TO PROTECT FLAVOR), NATURAL FLAVORS, PHOSPHORIC ACID, POTASSIUM SORBATE AND POTASSIUM BENZOATE (PRESERVE FRESHNESS), CARAMEL COLOR, ACESULFAME POTASSIUM, CALCIUM DISODIUM EDTA (TO PROTECT FLAVOR), RED 40.

With 150 calories, 10 teaspoons of added sugar, and a long list of artificial ingredients and colorings, this bottled iced tea has much more sugar than actual tea. So this iced tea is certainly not a healthy beverage, just a sugary drink.

Watch Out for Alcohol
The Lowdown on Beer, Wine, and Spirits

We've all heard about the heart health benefits of red wine. Red wine is a particularly rich source of antioxidant flavonoid phenolics, so many of the studies aiming to uncover the secret of red wine's effects have focused on its phenolic constituents, particularly resveratrol and the flavonoids. Resveratrol, found in grape skins and seeds, boosts HDL cholesterol and prevents blood clotting. Flavonoids, on the other hand, exhibit antioxidant properties that help prevent blood clots and plaque formation in arteries.

But red wine's potential heart health benefits do not warrant you to drink more, or to start drinking if you are a non-drinker! That's because studies have shown that drinking alcohol may increase triglycerides (a "bad" serum cholesterol) and is associated with increased cancer risk as well.

Need another compelling reason to go easy on alcohol? It is associated with weight gain. Researchers found that alcohol alters fat tissue metabolism, preventing it from oxidizing fat properly. This results in fat accumulation around the waist. Hello! Beer belly! This effect is exacerbated among infrequent drinkers, or people on a relatively higher-fat diet.[55] One gram of alcohol contains about seven calories—making it second only to fat in calorie density. In general, the higher the alcohol content in a drink, and the sweeter it is, the more calories it contains.

Beer
Regular beers, mostly lagers and ales, usually contain not more than 5% alcohol, with about 150 calories per 12-ounce serving.

Light beer usually contains less alcohol (about 4.2%) and fewer carbs, giving it a lighter taste and fewer calories at about 100 calories per 12-ounce serving.

Wine
White wine, which includes the full range of yellow and golden wines created from the juice of grapes that have the skins and seeds

removed just prior to fermentation, usually contains about 10–11% alcohol, and about 120 calories per five-ounce serving.

Red wines get their color from grapes with red and purple skins, and can range in color from bright red to near black. Like white wine, red wine contains about 10–11% alcohol, and it has just a few more calories: about 125 per 5-ounce serving.

When it comes to sparkling wine, Champagne is certainly the best known. It's simply a sparkling wine produced exclusively in the Champagne wine region of France. Most of the sparkling wines we drink are not actually Champagne, but blends of several grape varieties that go through a "secondary fermentation" that allows the gas that was released during the first fermentation to be reintroduced into the wine, giving the wine its characteristic bubbles. Sparkling wines, including Champagne, have fewer calories than red or white wine, at about 95 calories per five-ounce serving, but slightly more alcohol (about 12%).

Fortified wines like port and sherry are wines fortified with extra spirits. Among all wines, fortified wines are the highest in calories due to higher carb and alcohol contents. At more than 15% alcohol, fortified wine clocks in at more than 220 calories per five-ounce serving.

Coolers and Cocktails

Coolers and cocktails tend to be thought of as fun or feminine drinks—but they both pack quite a wallop when it comes to calories.

Alcoholic coolers have fancy, attractive labels, but you should always remember that they are still just alcoholic drinks. Like beer, alcoholic coolers have an alcohol content of about 5%. But coolers are often sweetened, so they contain more sugar, and therefore more calories, at about 225 calories per 12-ounce serving.

There are endless varieties of cocktails, of course, but they all have the same basic formula: one or more spirits mixed with sugar, syrup, juice, soda, milk, or some combination of these. A standard cocktail glass is 4.5 ounces, so standard-sized simple cocktails can come in under 200 calories per serving. However, we've seen more oversized cocktail glasses lately, from 6 ounces to even bigger ones like 12 ounces, so the calorie level of even a basic cocktail can easily balloon to 600–700 calories. If you're sipping a piña colada or daiquiri, you're consuming even more calories. A 4.5-ounce piña colada (with no maraschino cherries or other "goodies") has 245 calories, while a daiquiri has about 250. Of course, realistically, both of these drinks tend to be served in larger glasses, which bumps up the calorie count considerably.

Liquors and Liqueurs

Liquors, like rum, vodka, gin, and whiskey, have a higher alcohol content than wine or beer, and therefore have more calories per ounce. A 1.5-ounce serving of 80-proof liquor has 100–110 calories.

Liqueurs are usually liquors with cream and/or sugar added. The calorie level varies depending on what's added and the alcohol content. Based on 1.5-ounce servings, Grand Marnier has 112 calories, Irish cream liqueur like Bailey's has 154 calories, and coffee liqueur like Kahlua has 170 calories. Generally, liqueurs are high-sugar, high-alcohol drinks.

What's Really in Your Milk?

In the United States, conventional dairy cows are allowed to be injected with bovine growth hormones to beef up the milk supply. This often results in a condition called mastitis—an infection of the mammary glands. To prevent the infection, cows are routinely dosed with antibiotics. Don't like the idea of milk laced with growth hormone and antibiotics? Neither do I.

Organic Milk

The definition of "organic" when applied to milk is quite different from when it's applied to produce, because there are so many more factors involved when dealing with live animals. In addition to the cows being fed organic feed, USDA organic milk is produced by cows that have not been injected with bovine growth hormone or antibiotics, nor fed any animal by-products. The cows are also actively grazed on pasture and have access to the outdoors. Simply put, organic milk has no chemicals, pesticides, or hormones, and is produced by happy, healthy cows.

Goat's Milk

Goat's milk is another good alternative for those looking to avoid hormones and antibiotics. Since goat farming is a much smaller industry than that of dairy cows, goats tend to be raised on smaller farms in more natural conditions. Goats are not injected with growth hormone, because the bovine growth hormone doesn't work on goats, and the industry isn't large enough for anyone to have marketed a goat-specific growth hormone. Goat milk, with less lactose, can also be an option for those with mild lactose intolerance.

What About Cost?

Cost is the biggest reason why people are still willing to buy conventional milk, even if they don't like the idea of drinking growth hormone and antibiotics. That's because organic milk costs about twice as much as conventional milk. And goat's milk, while also free of hormones and antibiotics, costs twice as much as organic milk—four times as much as conventional cow's milk. If you're working with a limited budget, try to at least buy organic milk for your kids. Kids usually drink two to three cups of milk a day—quite

---

UnDiet Q&A: What about non-dairy milk?

These days, there's a milk to suit every preference, from those with lactose intolerance to those who prefer not to consume animal products. But how do almond milk, soy milk, hazelnut milk, rice milk, coconut milk, oat milk, and hemp milk stack up against dairy when in comes to nutrition and calcium content?

Although most non-dairy beverages are called "milk," they are naturally low in calcium. Some, but not all, have been fortified to offer a similar amount of calcium to cow's milk, but you can't assume. To be considered a good source of calcium, a product must contain at least 20% DV (daily value) of calcium per serving—so check the label if you're drinking a non-dairy milk to satisfy your calcium needs. Also check our Go UnDiet review to list milk that contains at least 20% DV of calcium. http://www.healthcastle.com/calciummilk.

Protein and calories are also quite varied. Rice milk contains the least amount of protein, at only 1 g per serving, while soy milk provides up to 11 g. Calories range from a low of 50–60 per cup for almond milk up to 140 for some brands of soy milk. Sweetened versions (like vanilla or chocolate flavors) usually add about four teaspoons of sugar in a serving. Choose unsweetened, plain, or original (slightly sweetened) versions instead.

In terms of fat, most non-dairy milks are low in fat to begin with, so light or fat-free versions are not necessary, and realistically save only 30 to 40 calories. Water and thickeners such as carrageenan are often added to dilute the calorie level in these light milks.

a bit more than most adults—and in their small bodies that's a lot. If you live in Canada, or near the Canadian border, you're in luck. That's because growth hormones and antibiotics are banned from use in dairy cows in Canada.

Should You Avoid Milk if You Can't Afford Organic?

Despite all the controversy about conventional milk, and the fact that most people really don't like the idea of drinking growth hormone and antibiotics, it's still better to drink some milk than avoid it altogether—even if you can't afford organic. That's because milk is the single highest source of calcium from food, and many of us don't get as much calcium as we should. Adults aged 19–50 need 1,000 mg of calcium a day, and one cup of milk provides about a third of that—290 mg of calcium. Also, milk has been found to be one of the top contributors of Vitamin D in the diets of children 2–18 years old (68.1% contribution to overall intake), as well as adults 19 years and older (46%).[56]

 Go UnDiet Action #27: Un-medicate your milk.
Buy organic milk whenever possible, especially if you're going to be serving it to your kids.

The Go UnDiet Formula for Healthy Drinks
The UnDiet Formula: 3+1

Not everyone drinks plain water all day, and that is totally fine. I don't expect to be able to do that myself, so I certainly don't expect it from others. Besides, some drinks are actually good for us. So my formula for healthy drinks is simply 3+1. What that means is that you should drink three calcium-containing drinks per day (dairy or non-dairy), plus one discretionary drink. The rest of your fluids should be plain water, or calorie-free tea or coffee. Besides, you should always think ahead about what you'll be drinking throughout the day. Most of us plan out what we'll eat for our three meals, so why don't you have a plan for your six to eight drinks a day?

So, how do you fit in three calcium-containing drinks? Certainly, drinking three cups of milk is the easiest way to get your three daily servings of calcium-containing drinks. If drinking milk straight up is not your cup of tea, then add it to your cup of tea. Adding milk to your tea or coffee, for instance, is another way many adults get their dairy. And Europeans certainly know that well. The French, Italian, and Spanish all have their own versions of their morning jolt of caffeine with a healthy serving of milk—cafe au lait, caffe latte, and cafe con leche, respectively!

Many non-dairy milks, like soy, almond, and hemp milk, are fortified with calcium. Refer to the Non-Dairy Milk sidebar on page 92 for more information and use the Go UnDiet Review Tool on my website http://www.healthcastle.com/product-listing .shtml?catid=9 to look for calcium-containing non-dairy milks.

What about OJ with added calcium?

I get asked this question a lot. My simple answer is that calcium-fortified orange juice should be your last resort. That's because milk offers a lot more than just calcium. Milk contains protein and Vitamin D, which cannot be found in OJ. Because of its protein and fat content, milk can actually make you feel fuller after drinking it, and hence may delay your hunger or decrease your intake at your next meal!

If you have lactose intolerance, try lactose-free milk. If you are a vegan or have a cow's milk protein allergy, try calcium-fortified non-dairy milk. Drink OJ with added calcium only if all other means to get your three calcium-containing drinks fail.

 Go UnDiet Action #28: Understand the UnDiet formula: 3+1.

Drink three servings of calcium-containing drinks, have up to one discretionary drink, and get the rest of your fluids from water, coffee, or tea.

One serving = 8 ounces

For your discretionary drink, if you really must drink something sweet, make sure it's something you really enjoy, rather than something you're just reaching for out of convenience. And, of course, the smaller the serving, the better. One serving is 8 ounces—anything more than that and you are getting into a second serving. Table 12 earlier in this chapter listed the calories for drinks based on 8-ounce servings. What you may not realize is that most of the drinks you buy in stores or in restaurants are much larger than eight ounces. One bottle of soda or iced tea is 20 ounces—that's 2.5 servings. The smallest frappuccino from Starbucks is 12 ounces, and the biggest is 24—so the largest frappuccino is actually three servings. At 7-11, the smallest slurpee is 12 ounces, while the biggest is 44—or 5.5 servings. And at Smoothie King, the smallest serving is 20 ounces (2.5 servings), while the largest is 40 ounces—or 5 servings!

All those super-sized drinks really pack in a shocking amount of calories.

Drink	Size	Calories
Rockstar Energy Drink	24 oz.	420
Starbucks White Hot Chocolate with 2% milk & whipped cream, venti	20 oz.	590
White Chocolate Crème Frappuccino blended beverage, Starbucks, with whole milk & whipped cream, venti	24 oz.	760
Smoothie King, Lemon Twist Strawberry, large	40 oz.	876
Chocolate Triple Thick Shake, McDonald's	32 oz.	1,160
Milkshake, Cold Stone's PB&C, Gotta Have It size	24 oz.	2,010

Table 13. Super-size (super-calorie) drinks

Seriously, a milkshake with over 2,000 calories? That's as many calories as most women should eat in an entire day! And while you may accept that you're getting a lot of calories when you're drinking a milkshake, you may not realize that over 400 calories are lurking in a can of energy drink.

Go UnDiet Action #29: Un-super-size your discretionary drinks.

Buy the smallest size possible—you're not really getting more bang for your buck with the larger size, you're just adding more inches to your waistline.

But Water is Boring!

It's true—water lacks that certain something. Most of us don't have a problem bringing water with us when we leave the house, and just about everyone has their own water bottle these days. But at a certain point, you may feel like you want something more than what's in your water bottle. When this urge strikes, you may have no choice but to head to a vending machine or convenience store, where sugary, super-sized drinks are really the only things on offer.

To prevent this scenario, and not be stuck with water that's boring your taste buds, keep a tea bag with you—either in your purse or your lunch bag. It doesn't really matter if it's tea with polyphenols (like we talked about earlier), or just an herbal tea with a flavor you enjoy. The important thing is that a simple tea bag gives you an easy, calorie-free way to liven up your water when you feel like you need something with a little taste.

If you're at home, or if your workplace has a freezer, you can also jazz up your water by adding frozen fruit. Just freeze any ripe fruit at home—cut-up berries, citrus wedges, melon balls, or peach puree—then use them as ice cubes. If you're at home, just drop them in your glass, or take a few to the office in a plastic bag. These colorful "ice cubes" really give life to boring water!

 Go UnDiet Action #30: Un-bore your water.
Use a tea bag or frozen fruit to add life to water, rather than reaching for sweetened drinks.

5 Small Steps to UnDiet

This chapter's Go UnDiet Actions are all about drinks. Your body needs fluids, but drinks can be a hidden source of sugar and calories, so use these small steps to work toward increasing your true water intake.

- ▶ **#26. Un-drink your calories.** Drinks are meant to hydrate us, not feed us, so they shouldn't be a big source of calories. Remember that calories from drinks don't make you feel full, so you don't eat any less food.

- ▶ **#27. Un-medicate your milk.** Buy organic whenever possible to avoid growth hormones and antibiotics.

- ▶ **#28. Understand the UnDiet formula: 3+1.** Drink three calcium-containing drinks per day (dairy or non-dairy) and have one discretionary drink if you need something sweet.

- ▶ **#29. Un-super-size your discretionary drinks.** A serving is 8 ounces. Look at the label of drinks you buy to see how many servings are really in each can or bottle.

- ▶ **#30. Un-bore your water.** Jazz up water with a tea bag or frozen fruit to make sure you get enough fluids without resorting to sugary drinks.

CHAPTER 7

Add Color and Carbs to Your Plate

If there's one food group that's misunderstood, it's carbs. With all the low-carb diets out there, and claims that carbs will make you fat, it's no wonder we're obsessed with this category of foods. But the truth is, it's unfair that carbs get such a bad rap. Potatoes and bagels are not the only carbs out there. In fact, all fruits and vegetables are considered carbs! All those anti-carb headlines may have scared us away from eating nutritious grains and root vegetables for a while, but now it's time to reclaim our carbs.

Will Carbs Make You Fat?
There's No Scientific Evidence that Carbs are Bad

Here's the simple truth. If you eat too much of any food group, you will gain weight—since gaining weight is a result of consuming more calories that you need. If you don't have diabetes, there is absolutely no scientific evidence that carbs in particular are bad for you or will cause you to gain weight.

If you go on a temporary diet (low-fat or low-carb), you will lose weight temporarily. There is no evidence to suggest that a low-carb diet is helpful beyond one year.[57] Some studies have even shown that it's only effective in losing weight for 6 months.[58]

So go ahead, reclaim your carbs. They are an essential part of any healthy eating plan.

Carbs Have Fewer Calories than Protein Foods

Despite everything you've heard about high-protein and low-carb diets, the fact is that carb foods actually have fewer calories by volume than any protein foods.

Food (1 cup)	Calories (kcal)
Veggies	
Spinach, raw	7
Romaine lettuce, shredded	8
Tomato, chopped	32
Broccoli, chopped	31
Carrot, chopped	52
Potato, baked, without salt	113
Fruit	
Apple, chopped, with skin	65
Strawberries, sliced	53
Blueberries, whole	84
Cantaloupe, balls	60
Honeydew melon, balls	64

Meat	
Pork tenderloin, roasted	338
Chicken thigh, roasted	293
Tuna, canned in water	179
Tuna, canned in oil	289
Ground beef, pan-broiled	566
Sirloin beef, roasted	462
Nuts/Beans	
Peanuts, raw	828
Mixed nuts, dry roasted	814
Walnuts, English, shelled	654
Kidney beans, canned	215
Baked beans, canned, no salt added	266
Grains	
White rice, cooked	205
Brown rice, cooked	216
Spaghetti, whole wheat, cooked	174
Spaghetti, enriched, without added salt	221

Table 14. Calories in carb foods and protein foods
Source: USDA

Your stomach can only hold a certain volume of food, but that volume of food can vary wildly when it comes to the amount of calories. Think about it this way: **One cup of veggies on your plate has at least five times fewer calories than an equal volume of meat.**

Add More Color to Your Plate
How Many Servings of Fruit and Vegetables Do You Need Per Day?

How many veggies?

Average Adult Female: 2.5–3 servings

Average Adult Male: 3–4 servings

How much fruit?

Average Adult Female: 1.5–2 servings

Average Adult Male: 2–2.5 servings

So what's a serving? Take a look at Table 15 below for a simple explanation.

Food	Amount to Equal One Serving
Fruit	One cup, cut up
Raw vegetables	Two cups
Cooked vegetables	One cup

Table 15. Serving sizes for fruits and vegetables

Now, I know what you're thinking after looking at the serving size for raw vegetables: How on earth are you supposed to eat that much salad every day? The key is not to focus on salad! Yes, you should eat some raw vegetables, but remember that cooked vegetables count too—and the serving size is half as big. Go and get a measuring cup and take a look at how big one cup really is. Think about that cup filled with cooked broccoli or carrots. It's really not that much at all. I can easily eat 1.5–2 cups of cooked vegetables at every meal, and, once you get into the habit, you will be able to do so too. Regardless of the amount, start by adding some produce to every meal—including breakfast. Throw some strawberries or bananas in your cereal, or have a fruit smoothie. At lunch, munch on some carrot or celery sticks. And at dinner, explore new ways to cook with vegetables. We'll talk more about some ways to spice up your cooked vegetables later in this section.

Count Colors Instead of Servings

Now that you know how much produce you should be eating, I want to let you in on a secret. It's actually more important to eat a wide variety of colorful fruits and vegetables every day than it is to count your servings. The best way to get a real variety of nutrients from your fruits and vegetables is to choose items from several different color groups. The science has shown that there are huge benefits to mixing and matching our produce colors. That's because each color contains different sets of phytochemicals that provide different health benefits.

There are many more vegetables out there than lettuce and tomatoes! I often talk about variety. And it is more than avoiding monotony. As Table 16 shows, different color groups are rich in different antioxidants, offering extra health bonuses. Indeed, a study[59] found that a diversified variety of fruit and vegetables is linked to lower risk of certain cancers.

Color	Fruits	Vegetables	Benefits
Red	• red apples • watermelon • pink grapefruit • cherries • cranberries, strawberries & raspberries • rhubarb • red grapes	• red bell peppers • tomatoes • beets • red cabbage • red potatoes • radishes	Lycopene shows promise in fighting lung and prostate cancers, and anthocyanins are powerful antioxidants that may help prevent heart disease.
Purple	• concord grapes & raisins • blueberries & blackberries • plums & prunes • figs	• eggplant	Anthocyanins may help ward off heart disease by preventing clot formation. They may also help lower the risk of cancer.
Green	• green apples • green grapes • honeydew melon • kiwi • limes	• spinach • broccoli • brussels sprouts • bok choy • artichokes • avocados • asparagus • green beans • green cabbage • cucumbers • lettuce • green onions • peas • green pepper	Lutein appears to reduce the risk of heart disease and stroke as well as guard against age-related macular degeneration. Dark green leafy vegetables are usually high in folate, a B vitamin that shows promising results in preventing heart diseases. In addition, sulforaphane, a phytochemical present in cruciferous vegetables, has been found to detoxify cancer-causing chemicals before they damage the body.

Orange	• mango • oranges • yellow apples • apricots • cantaloupe • yellow grapefruit • lemons • peaches	• pumpkin • carrots • butternut squash • yellow peppers • rutabagas • corn • sweet potatoes	Beta carotenes may help prevent cancer, particularly of the lung, esophagus, and stomach. They may also reduce the risk of heart disease and improve immune function.
White	• bananas	• cauliflower • mushrooms • onions • potatoes • turnips	Anthoxanthins and allicin can help lower blood pressure and protect against stomach cancer.

Table 16. Examples of fruits and vegetables in each color group

Go UnDiet Action #31: Un-count 5-a-day and count 3-a-day instead.

Instead of the old 5-a-day slogan, which referred to servings, focus on eating fruits and vegetables from three different color groups each day. And remember to eat some produce at every meal!

Make Vegetables a Main Dish

At mealtime, vegetables tend to be relegated to side-dish status. But there's no reason vegetables can't be a main dish. I always plan my dinner around what vegetables I have in the house. So how do you promote veggies to being your dinner's star attraction? You need to think outside the box and apply real cooking techniques to your vegetables, just like you would to your meat.

Remember: Salad is not the only way to get your veggies. Opening up a bag of pre-prepared salad and drizzling some dressing on is certainly easy—but it's boring, and that bagged salad is never going to become the centerpiece of a meal. So here are three easy ways to brighten up your veggies and make them main-course-worthy.

Veggie Cooking Tip #1: Just like you season other dishes, season your veggies!

When we cook meat, pasta, and other dishes, we use seasonings. Yet, for some reason, people seem afraid to experiment with seasoning their vegetables. But eating vegetables is not meant to be a punishment—so it's okay to make them taste good! I like to add flavor to cooked veggies by using butter and adding herbs like basil, parsley, dill, roasted garlic, oregano, grated ginger, and so on. You can also try adding a citrus flavor to veggies by squeezing in some orange or lemon juice, or adding grated orange or lemon rind to butter or olive oil to make a tasty dressing.

If you want to add flavor in the simplest way possible, try using some of the sauces you already have around the house—like soy sauce, peanut sauce, or miso—or throw on some sesame seeds or nuts for added crunch. Anything you can use to season meat, you can use to season vegetables, so don't be afraid to experiment. You'll be surprised how just a little bit of seasoning can turn those "boring" vegetables into something really delicious!

One more tip on seasoning vegetables—and this one works especially well if you have kids. Try sprinkling some natural cheese on top of cooked vegetables. It's a simple way to make them richer, and much more appealing to kids.

Veggie Cooking Tip #2: Use different cooking methods for different vegetables

Sure, you can boil carrots. But there are many more ways to cook vegetables, and knowing which method best suits the vegetable you're using and the kind of flavor you're trying to achieve can really make a difference.

Root vegetables, like yams, sweet potatoes, and turnips, are excellent for roasting. Summer favorites like corn on the cob, bell peppers, and asparagus work really well on the grill. And stir-frying is a great way to cook vegetables if you're in a hurry. So don't limit yourself to boiling!

Of course, some vegetables, like butter lettuce, baby spinach, some brightly-colored peppers, and especially baby tomatoes, are naturally sweet and are best enjoyed uncooked. Throw these in your salads instead of just sticking to that bagged salad mix.

Veggie Cooking Tip #3: Add sweetness

Some people find green and white vegetables to be bitter. The good news is, it's easy to sweeten them up. If you're serving these vegetables raw, try adding fresh or dried fruits. The natural sweetness of the fruit helps to balance out the bitterness, and adds great texture to salads. If you're cooking these vegetables, try adding a drizzle of maple syrup or honey—these natural sweeteners balance out the bitterness without overwhelming the taste of the vegetables.

When I stir-fry or steam green vegetables, I always add just a pinch of sugar when the vegetables are half-cooked. Not only does it add a little bit of sweetness, sugar actually helps the green vegetables stay a nice bright green.

Go UnDiet Action #32: Un-side your veggies!
Once they're dressed up a bit with some seasonings, new cooking techniques, or a bit of sweetness, veggies can become an excellent main dish. Don't be afraid to experiment with new flavors!

Bring on the Beans

So far in this chapter, we've focused on adding color to your plate by eating more vegetables. But beans can add red, black, yellow, and white colors to your plate as well.

Beans don't get a lot of attention in American cooking. Other than vegetarians or those cooking up a batch of chili for a tailgate party, not too many people give beans the attention they deserve. Partly, this is because beans are just not that glamorous. But it's also partly because beans tend to suffer from an identity crisis. So let's clear one thing up right now—beans, believe it or not, are actually vegetables.

Forget the Identity Crisis—Beans are Vegetables

Yes, it's true. Beans are vegetables. I can't blame you if you're surprised it's this simple, since beans tend to get lumped into other food groups. Some people consider beans to be a meat substitute or a plant-based protein. Sometimes they're called "legumes, lentils, and pulses," and sometimes they're even lumped in with nuts and seeds. But beans are not meat substitutes or nuts! They are vegetables. You'll find them under the vegetables category on the MyPyramid dietary guidelines.

A recent study showed we only eat 0.1 cups of cooked dried beans and peas a day,[60] while the Dietary Guidelines recommend we eat 3 cups of legumes per week. Of course, there's that word "legumes" again. Since most people can't give an accurate definition of legumes, why don't we just call them beans? Everyone knows what beans are! Once you understand that when you see the word "legumes" you can just mentally cross it out and substitute beans, you'll see that the Dietary Guidelines recommend that we eat four times more beans than we are eating now. And there are many more beans available than the old pork-and-beans from a can your mom used to serve. Here's a list of some common beans to keep an eye out for at the grocery store.

Common Types of Beans

adzuki	garbanzo beans (chickpeas)	pinto beans
black beans	kidney beans	soybeans
black-eyed peas	lima beans	white beans
cranberry beans	navy beans	

 Go UnDiet Action #33: Un-complicate your beans.
Beans are an easy way to add color to your plate, and they count as vegetables. It doesn't need to be any more complicated than that!

No Time to Cook Beans? Don't Worry!

Does the prep work involved in eating beans scare you away? Don't worry. You don't always need an overnight soak to get rid of the gas associated with eating beans! Try one of the three methods below to speed up your bean prep time and make it easier to incorporate these important vegetables into your meals.

Bean Cooking Method #1: Quick Soak

Nutrition consultant Robyn Flipse, MS, RD suggests a quick soak method. Put beans and water in a pot and bring to a boil. Turn off the heat and let sit for an hour, then rinse.

Bean Cooking Method #2: Use Canned or Frozen Beans

Both canned and frozen beans have been pre-soaked, rinsed, and pre-cooked. Edamame, for instance, is usually available in frozen format. Simply boil or microwave for immediate enjoyment. For canned beans, Flipse recommends purchasing no-added-flavor varieties. Remember, even with no-salt-added varieties, it's best to rinse all canned beans before using.

Bean Cooking Method #3: Pressure Cooker

Did you receive a pressure cooker at your wedding or as a house-warming gift? It's time to bring it out from the dusty storage area. Making beans in a pressure cooker significantly cuts cooking time and should be as easy as 1-2-3. Jill Nussinow, author of the instructional pressure cooker DVD *Pressure Cooking: A Fresh Look at Delicious Dishes in Minutes* shares these foolproof tips:

- *Step 1:* After rinsing pre-soaked beans, simply add half a cup of water for every cup of beans, and mix with other ingredients in the cooker.

- *Step 2:* Cook beans for 6 to 10 minutes until the cooker comes to pressure. Turn the heat down low to maintain the pressure for about 10 minutes.

- *Step 3:* Turn off the heat and let it sit. Wait for the cooker to be ready.

Don't Fear Frozen and Canned
Fresh May Be Best, But Frozen and Canned Count, Too

Nothing beats the taste, texture, and appearance of fresh produce, but the simple fact is that it can be difficult to keep fresh produce on hand through the week. The good news is that frozen and canned produce offer the same health benefits as the fresh stuff, but are much easier to purchase ahead of time and store. In fact, in 1998, the Food & Drug Administration (FDA) confirmed that frozen fruits and vegetables provide the same essential nutrients and health benefits as fresh. That's because frozen fruits and vegetables are nothing more than fresh fruits and vegetables that have been blanched (cooked for a short time in boiling water or steamed) and frozen within hours of being picked. And canned produce has similar nutrition to fresh or frozen. Further, frozen and canned fruits and vegetables are processed at their peak in terms of freshness and nutrition. On days you run out of fresh produce, frozen and canned versions are your best bets for an easy way to get some fruit and vegetables into your meals.

Of course, even if you haven't run out of fresh produce, there are times when you may want to use frozen or canned versions—just because it's easier. That's totally okay, too! For example, frozen produce is always pre-washed and pre-cut, which can make it much easier to use in recipes that would otherwise involve a lot of chopping. Frozen squash is much easier to use than fresh squash if you're making soup, pasta filling, or any recipe that calls for a pureed or mashed texture, since the squash is already peeled and cut, and soft from the pre-freeze blanching. And while nothing beats the sweet, juicy taste of fresh berries, frozen berries work great in baking or in sauces when fresh berries are not in season.

When it comes to cans, my pantry is always stocked with plenty of no-salt-added canned beans. Canned beans are much softer than dried, of course, so they don't work as well in dishes that call for a firm bean texture, but they are perfect for mashed dishes like dip, or to throw in a salad.

Simply put, all forms of produce count—fresh, frozen, and canned. So when you're thinking about getting your three colors for the day (as discussed in Go UnDiet Action #31), don't forget to check your pantry and freezer for some extra options. Making a dish from a can of beans may not be a glamorous culinary adventure, but it is a much better option than a fried chicken dinner with fries, or a greasy pizza, or any number of other easy but not-very-good-for-you options.

Go UnDiet Action #34: Un-focus on fresh.
Fresh produce may have the best taste, texture, and appearance, but sometimes frozen or canned produce is just easier to fit into your day. Canned and frozen produce are full of the same nutritional benefits as the fresh stuff, so fit them into your meals to add some healthy nutritional punch to your plate.

What About Organic?
Why Buy Organic Produce?

The main benefit of organic produce is that it has not been exposed to pesticides. This is a big benefit—after all, who likes the idea of pesticides in their food? And the idea has certainly caught on. Organic food is a $25 billion industry. To be exact, in 2009, $24.8 billion worth of organic food was sold in the United States alone.[61] Organic fruits and vegetables represented 38% of total organic food sales, an 11.4% increase from 2008. What's important for you to know is that the label "organic" refers to the way the produce is grown—it does not indicate the final quality of the produce. In fact, there's been an ongoing debate about whether organic food is any more nutritious, but the answer seems to be no (see the sidebar for more information).

Still, even if science doesn't show that there are any nutritional advantages to eating organic produce, I believe that you are what you eat. The same goes for plants—so those that are grown in an organic, natural setting that's free from pesticides are much more appealing to me. Improved nutrition is not the main reason people buy organics—most people buy organic food because of a concern about pesticides or the environmental impact of non-organic farming methods, as well as the taste. In her book *Cool Cuisine*, chef Laura Stec said, "growing plants in carbon-rich soil is like simmering them in the best Bordelaise sauce you've ever made." For me it's about taste, too. Personally, I love bananas. I can eat a banana every single day, because it's so easy—all I have to do is peel it and eat it! I tried an organic banana years ago, and it tasted so much better than regular bananas that I've been buying organic fruit ever since.

Make the Most of Your Organic Food Budget

While many people like the idea of buying organic produce, it can often be just too expensive. If you're working with a limited food budget and can't afford to buy all your produce organic, use the following strategies to maximize your organic intake.

UnDiet Q&A: Is organic produce more nutritious?

Recent studies have shown no difference in nutrient content between organic and non-organic produce. A 2009 literature review by the French Agency for Food Safety (AFSSA) reported no difference in mineral content between organic and conventionally grown fruit.[62] Another 2009 systematic review commissioned by the UK's Food Safety Association looked at all studies published since 1958. The researchers found no evidence that organic produce is more nutritious than conventionally grown produce.[63] Of course, no one has ever suggested that organic produce is any less nutritious, either. So don't give up on organic produce, even though science hasn't proved that it is more nutritious.

1. Choose organic for unpeeled fruits: When you peel a fruit, you remove many of the pesticides. Focus on buying organic for fruits you won't peel, like berries, apples, grapes, and peaches.

2. Choose organic for the Dirty Dozen: Every year, the Environmental Working Group (EWG) publishes a list of the top-12 worst offenders when it comes to pesticides. This year's list includes celery, peaches, strawberries, apples, blueberries, nectarines, bell peppers, spinach, kale, cherries, potatoes, and imported grapes. You can find the list at http://www.foodnews.org/EWG-shoppers-guide-download-final.pdf.

3. Buy seasonal organic produce: The price difference of organic versus conventionally-grown produce is 10%–20% when in season. If the produce is not in season, it costs a lot more. For instance, blueberries are in season in the summertime. In February, I bought some organic blueberries from Chile, and the price was almost double. To find out what's in season, go to http://www.fruitsand veggiesmorematters.org/?page_id=674.

4. Visit a farmers' market: Local farmers usually use organic techniques to grow their produce, even though they may not have an organic certification. (Official organic certification can be too expensive for local farmers with smaller crops.) Local produce also retains more nutrients, because it's fresher. And since there are fewer transport costs, local organic produce generally costs less than organic food brought in from afar (and it's better for the environment, too). Plus, you won't find any highly processed foods to tempt you at a farmers' market! According to the USDA, in 2008 there were close to 4,700 farmers markets operating across the United States. Chances are you will be able to find one fairly close to where you live. Check LocalHarvest.org and EatWellGuide .org for locations.

5. Join a CSA: CSA stands for community-supported agriculture, and it provides a way for urbanites to get access to farm-fresh produce. In a CSA, the consumer purchases a share (usually by prepaying a set amount of money to the farm or farmer) at the beginning of the growing season. This allows the farmer to purchase seeds and any other growing equipment needed. In exchange, the member will receive locally-grown/produced, ultra-fresh foods with maximum flavor and vitamin benefits throughout the growing season as the crops are harvested. But farm-fresh local produce is not the only benefit of joining a CSA. Most CSAs allow consumers who purchase shares to visit the farm at least once per season. This allows you to develop a relationship with the farmer who grows your food, and learn more about how food is grown. Kids also get a kick out of farm visits, and are typically more willing to eat produce from "their" farm—even veggies they've never been known to eat before! Plus, you will get exposed to new vegetables and ways of cooking you might never have thought to try.

Some CSAs will deliver the crops to members' homes, while others will deliver to a pick-up depot. Both LocalHarvest.org/csa and EatWellGuide.org provide searchable directories of farms that offer CSA shares for purchase. Having a constant supply of fresh produce will give you no excuse for not eating fruits and vegetables!

6. Grow your own: The ultimate commitment to eating local food is to learn to grow some of your own. This doesn't mean having to farm acres of land or raising livestock; even container gardening (with herbs) is a good starting point. If you are completely new to it, grow only a few select plants that you know your family will eat, and seek out lots of advice from experienced gardeners among your family or friends. There are also many gardening sources on the web. For example, GardenABCs.com provides multiple resources for parents and teachers to get started and maintain school gardens. A site out of the UK, GrowVeg.com, provides lots of free articles on common gardening questions. And, of course, check out the cooperative extension program at your local university for free publications or fact sheets on food gardening. Many universities or colleges also offer gardening workshops or classes to the community.

Go UnDiet Action #35: Un-expense your organics budget.

You can reduce your pesticide intake without spending a fortune buying all-organic produce. Use the tips in this chapter to maximize your organic budget and reduce the amount of pesticides you consume.

5 Small Steps to UnDiet

This chapter's Go UnDiet Actions are all about adding more color to your plate. As you plan your family's meals over the next few weeks, focus on adding more color to each and every meal.

▶ **#31. Un-count 5-a-day and count 3-a-day instead.** Instead of focusing on getting 5 servings per day, aim for three colors a day and eat produce at every meal.

▶ **#32. Un-side your veggies.** One sure way to get more vegetables in your diet is to promote them from side dish to main course.

▶ **#33. Un-complicate your beans.** Remember, beans are vegetables—and they can add lots of color to any meal.

▶ **#34. Un-focus on fresh.** Frozen and canned produce offer the same nutritional benefits as the fresh stuff, and are easier to keep on hand. Make sure to stock your freezer and pantry with frozen and canned fruits and vegetables so you can eat well even if you don't have time for a mid-week grocery run.

▶ **#35. Un-expense your organics budget.** You don't need to buy all-organic produce to reduce your intake of pesticides. Focus on the strategies in this chapter to make the most of your organics budget.

CHAPTER 8

Watch Out for the Extras

Drinking calories is the number-one reason why we are overweight. Overeating is the second reason. The third reason is all the little extras we pile onto our foods. So let's take a look at where all those "extras" creep into the foods we eat, and how we can avoid the extra calories they add each day.

Don't Blame the Carbs—Blame the Toppings

Carbs, like breads, potatoes, pasta, bagels, and so on, are often blamed for making us fat. We all know someone who's on a low-carb/no-carb diet. But if you look carefully, the problem is not the carbs themselves, but the fact that we tend to pile high-calorie extras on top of our carbs.

Carb food	Serving Size	Calories	Total Fat (g)	Carbs (g)	Sodium (mg)
Baked potato	1 serving (6 oz.)	158	0	36	17
Baked potato with toppings	1 serving	389	17	39	1,296
Pasta, plain	1 serving	390	4	79	260
Alfredo pasta	1 serving	1,000	63	88	1,220
Bagel, plain	1 bagel	260	1.5	52	450
Bagel with cream cheese	1 serving	361	11.5	52.8	536
Bread	1 slice (0.9 oz.)	67	0.8	12.7	160
Bread with butter	1 serving	271	23.8	12.7	324

Table 17. Carbs vs. carbs plus toppings

As you can see, carbs themselves are not so bad. But the extras we pile on can double or even triple the calories, and exponentially increase the amount of fat. It's not the carbs that are making us fat—it's the bacon and cheese we put on our baked potatoes, the alfredo sauce we put on our pasta, and the cream cheese we slather on our bagels!

Go UnDiet Action #36: Un-blame carbs and blame the extras instead.

Sure, extras add a bit of flavor, but they add a ton of extra calories and fat.

Our Obsession with Dip

As a culture, we've developed many small, daily habits that contribute to our calorie banks, and we may not even realize it. For example, we are obsessed with sauces, dressings, and dips! Many menu items come with sauces and dips—fries, salad, fish, bread sticks, chicken nuggets, and even already-saucy hot wings are all served with extra sauce or dips. But the one that really gets me is pizza. Most pizza-delivery restaurants now offer free dips with each pizza. But do we really need to dip a pizza that's covered in sauce and cheese into a dip?

So just how many calories can a little sauce or dip actually add to a snack or a meal? You might be surprised.

Sauce, Dressing, or Dip	Size	Calories	Fat (g)	Carb (g)	Sodium (mg)
Soy sauce	1 packet (2 tsp/12g)	7	0	0.7	670
Ketchup	2 packets	30	0	6	220
Sweet & sour sauce for nuggets	1 pack	50	0	12	120
Spicy Buffalo sauce	1 pack (1.3 oz.)	60	6	1	800
Caramel dip for apples in kids' meals	1 pack (21 g)	70	0.5	15	35
Miracle Whip, regular	1 oz.	80	7	4	210
Caramel sauce for BK apple fries	2 packs (28 g)	90	1	20	70

Cheez Whiz, regular	1 oz.	90	7	4	440
Honey mustard sauce for nuggets	1 pack	130	12	6	220
Caesar dressing, Kraft	2 Tbsp	130	12	2	380
Ranch dressing, Hidden Valley	2 Tbsp	140	14	2	280
Creamy ranch sauce	1 packet (1.3 oz.)	170	18	2	270
Tartar sauce	1 packet (1 oz.)	190	38	2	30
Creamy Caesar dressing	1 packet (2 oz.)	190	18	4	500
Blue cheese dipping cup	1 dipping cup (1.5 oz.)	240	25	2	310
Garlic dipping cup	1 dipping cup (1 oz.)	250	28	0	160

Table 18. Calories, fat, carbs, and sodium in sauces, dressings, and dips

As you can see, a little soy sauce won't add too many calories to a meal (although it does add a lot of sodium), but just one of those garlic dips that comes with pizza these days adds 250 calories and 28 grams of fat to what's already a high-calorie, high-fat meal.

 Go UnDiet Action #37: Un-dip finger foods.
Many finger foods are high in calories to begin with, so why add even more by dipping them in sauce?

UnDiet Q&A: What's in your cheese?

You may have heard that all the cheese we pile on our food these days is a big culprit in our obesity epidemic. But you really shouldn't be afraid of cheese. If you cover a whole pizza with a layer of cheese, certainly it's high in calories! But when used properly, a small amount of cheese adds flavor and aroma no other condiments can offer. So don't write off flavorful cheese, simply use it like you use herbs—that is, in small amounts!

To make cheese, only four ingredients are needed: milk, culture, enzymes, and salt. These are the ingredients you'll find in natural cheese. Processed cheese, on the other hand, may be loaded with ingredients like coloring agents, sodium phosphates, maltodextrin, carrageenan, cellulose gum, lactic acid, citric acid, sorbic acid, etc.

Watch Out for Added Sugar
Do You Know How Much Sugar You Consume?

You'll probably be shocked when I tell you that the average American adult consumes 22 teaspoons of added sugar per day, and the average American teenager consumes 34 teaspoons. Just picture what that would look like spooned into a coffee cup! Studies have shown a link between added sugar and increased body weight and body fat.[64] It's no wonder that the American Heart Association recommends a drastic cut in the amount of added sugar we consume, down to six teaspoons for women and nine teaspoons for men.

You may think that you couldn't possibly consume 22 teaspoons of sugar a day. Whenever I mention this number, people's jaws drop with disbelief, and they always tell me that there's no way they consume that much sugar. But do you know how much sugar you are really consuming every day? Do you know where sugar is lurking? You may think that a slice of chocolate cake or a candy bar is the biggest source of sugar in your day, but the truth is that most of the sugar we consume is lurking in drinks. Take a look at the sugar content of some of these common drinks and foods.

Drink	Serving Size	Sugar (tsp.)
Slurpee, large	40 oz.	21 tsp
Regular soda, bottle	20 oz.	13 tsp
Regular iced tea, bottle	20 oz.	10 tsp
Ben & Jerry's All-Natural Chocolate ice cream	1 cup	10 tsp
Regular soda, can	12 oz.	8 tsp
Vitaminwater, bottle	20 oz.	8 tsp
Iced cappuccino, small	12 oz.	7.5 tsp
Slurpee, small	12 oz.	6.5 tsp
Kit Kat	1 bar	5 tsp
Yoplait Whips yogurt	4 oz.	5 tsp
Haagen-Dazs ice cream bar with chocolate coating	1 bar	4.5 tsp
Kellogg's Honey Smacks cereal	1 cup	4.5 tsp

Table 19. High-sugar drinks and foods

You may be surprised to see that a bottle of iced tea has as much added sugar as a cup of ice cream, or that a bottle of Vitaminwater actually has more sugar than a Kit Kat candy bar. When you take a look at these numbers, it's easy to see how we end up consuming 22 teaspoons of added sugar every day.

The worst part is that 22 teaspoons of added sugar equals 370 extra empty calories every day, just from added sugar that doesn't even make us feel full. That leads me to point out one very compelling reason to cut your sugar intake from 22 teaspoons to 6 teaspoons a day—it will help save 270 calories a day!

Check Your Drinks

Before you get stressed out about looking for hidden sugar in your foods, take a look at your drinks. You can see from Table 19 that sweetened drinks have a ton of sugar. In fact, most of our daily empty calories come from drinks. We get an average of 450 to 550 calories per day from drinks—and a 2007 study found that 60% of those calories are from sweetened drinks like soda, flavored drinks, sports drinks, sweetened (flavored) milk, and so on.[65] Still not convinced? Harvard researchers reviewed 30 studies and found an association between drinking sugar-sweetened drinks and weight gain, in both adults and kids.[66]

This doesn't mean that a little bit of sugar is going to make you gain weight, but it certainly indicates a lifestyle trend. People who drink soda on a regular basis likely have a different lifestyle from people who, say, shop at farmers' markets every weekend. So, I'm not trying to tell you that you can never put sugar in your drinks to add flavor. Most people put about two teaspoons of sugar in their coffee. That's nothing alarming. But would you add 21 teaspoons of sugar to a glass of water? That's how much sugar there is in a bottle of orange soda—and that is exactly how we get to an average of 22 teaspoons of sugar per day.

 Go UnDiet Action #38: Un-sweeten your drinks.
A couple of teaspoons of sugar in your coffee is okay, but remember that a can of soda contains 8 teaspoons of sugar and a bottle contains 13 teaspoons.

Should You Go for Artificial Sweeteners?

If added sugar is something to cut down on, should you switch to using artificial sweeteners instead? First, let's clarify exactly what we mean by artificial sweeteners.

Sweetener	Brand	Year Approved For Use in Foods
Saccharin	Sweet 'N Low, Sweet Twin, Sugar Twin	1977
Aspartame	Equal, NutraSweet, NatraTaste	1981
Acesulfame-K	Sweet One, Sunett	1988
Sucralose	Splenda	1998
Neotame	Neotame	2002
Steviol glycosides	Sun Crystals, PureVia, Truvia, Stevia Extract in the Raw, Sweet Leaf	2009

Table 20. Artificial sweeteners at a glance
Source: *The American Journal of Clinical Nutrition*[67]

As you can see, there are quite a few options when it comes to artificial sweeteners. So, can they solve the added-sugar problem? To answer that question, let's talk about the case of diet soda, which is one of the most common ways people consume artificial sweeteners.

Is Diet Soda Better than Regular Soda?

Researchers from Boston University studied data from more than 6,000 middle-aged adults participating in a large-scale study called the Framingham Heart Study. These participants were all free of metabolic syndrome—a cluster of symptoms such as excessive fat around the waist, impaired fasting glucose, high blood pressure, low levels of "good" HDL cholesterol, and more—when the study started. After four years of follow up, researchers found that adults who drank one or more sodas a day (diet *or* regular) had about a 50 percent higher risk of having metabolic syndrome.[68]

Prior studies had linked the consumption of regular soda and its high levels of sugar with multiple risk factors for heart disease, but the Framingham study was the first to find that the link extends to low-calorie, artificially sweetened diet soda. The most intriguing finding of the study was that participants who drank one or more sodas per day—again, regular *or* diet—had a 31 percent greater risk of becoming overweight. The results surprised the researchers, who expected to see a difference between weight gain in regular and diet soda drinkers. Researchers observed a few possible reasons for their findings—one being that people who drink any kind of soda on a regular basis tend to have similar diet patterns: a diet with higher calories, saturated and trans fat, lower fiber and dairy, and a sedentary lifestyle.

So, the simple answer is no. Diet soda is not a healthy alternative to regular soda, even though it does not contain added sugar. If you're currently a soda addict, it's a much better option to find ways to slowly kick the habit rather than simply switching to diet soda.

What About Other Uses of Artificial Sweeteners?

Studies are not conclusive about whether artificial sweeteners actually help you lose weight or eat fewer calories. In fact, studies on rats have actually suggested that artificial sweeteners may promote weight gain, likely because you tend to compensate for the reduced calories in artificially sweetened foods by overeating other foods.[69] There is epidemiological support for the fact that artificially sweetened beverages lead to weight gain in children.[70] And, what's worse, some studies have found that artificial sweeteners in non-energy foods like chewing gum, flavored water, diet drinks, and other zero-calorie drinks can actually increase hunger.[71]

UnDiet Q&A: Is fructose really bad?

In recent years, high fructose corn syrup (HFCS) has been singled out and suggested to be linked to our obesity crisis. It's been targeted because soda has become our primary source of sugar, and HFCS is the main sugar used in soda (and soda's main source of calories). This soda connection has led some people to connect HFCS directly with obesity.

The fallout is that some people have become obsessed with fructose—obsessed, that is, with avoiding it. Manufacturers have definitely caught on to this consumer trend. Many have announced that they are phasing out HFCS and are switching back to "real sugar"—by which they mean regular white sugar (which is 100% sucrose). Some companies have gone even further. Pepsi, for instance, introduced Pepsi Natural, made with sugar instead of HFCS.[72]

INGREDIENTS (PEPSI NATURAL): SPARKLING WATER, SUGAR, NATURAL APPLE EXTRACT (COLOR), CARAMEL COLOR, CITRIC ACID, CAFFEINE, ACACIA GUM, TARTARIC ACID, LACTIC ACID, NATURAL FLAVOR, KOLA NUT EXTRACT.

INGREDIENTS (REGULAR PEPSI): CARBONATED WATER, HIGH FRUCTOSE CORN SYRUP, CARAMEL COLOR, SUGAR, PHOSPHORIC ACID, CAFFEINE, CITRIC ACID, NATURAL FLAVOR.

The main difference between these two products is the use of sugar instead of HFCS in Pepsi Natural. But simply switching from fructose to sucrose doesn't really solve the problem—and it certainly won't help you lose weight. A junk food made with "real" sugar instead of HFCS is still a junk food! It's still got 150 calories per can.

In fact, fructose is not unnatural at all. It's called fructose because it's naturally found in fruits! So, don't be fearful of fructose in particular, and don't be fooled into thinking that other sugar options are somehow healthier.

Go UnDiet Action #39: Un-fake your sugar.
Unless you have diabetes, stay clear of artificial sweeteners, which are usually found in foods and drinks with empty calories anyway.

Is Natural Sugar Better?

With all the concern about added sugars, some manufacturers are now marking their products as natural, organic, raw, or as having low GI (glycemic index). The fact is, all of these sugars—as well as plain old refined white sugar—are from natural sources. They are just refined to different degrees. Refining changes the taste profile, but nutrition-wise they are all the same. All of these sugars are made from sugar cane or sugar beet—and since neither sugar cane nor sugar beet has much nutritional value to begin with, the level of refining is not going to change the fact that sugar is simply not a nutritious food.

When you're trying to figure out the difference between different types of sugar, keep in mind that white sugar is simply sugar cane or sugar beet refined to be 100% sucrose. Molasses is what's left over after the white sugar is refined. And brown sugar is just white sugar with some molasses added. Sugar goes by many different names these days, so watch out for any of the following terms on an ingredients list when you're trying to figure out how much added sugar a product really contains.

- white sugar
- brown sugar
- icing sugar
- invert sugar
- maple syrup
- honey
- molasses
- brown rice syrup

- corn syrup
- high fructose corn syrup
- cane juice
- evaporated cane juice
- all fruit juice concentrates, including apple and pear
- all "ose" ingredients including dextrose, fructose, lactose, glucose, maltose and sucrose

The important thing to remember is that all sugars contain similar calories, and are metabolized by the body similarly, whether the sugar is natural or not. All sugars contain between 15 and 21 calories per teaspoon, as you can see in Table 21.

Type of Sugar	Calories (per tsp)
Natural cane sugar	15
Sugar, granulated	17
Sugar, brown (packed)	17
Maple syrup	17
High fructose corn syrup	18
Molasses	19
Agave nectar	19
Honey	21
Corn syrup, light	21

Table 21. Calories in sugar

Go UnDiet Action #40: Un-source your sugar.
Natural, raw, brown, white—all kinds of sugar have similar calories. Limit your intake of added sugar to six teaspoons per day, whether the sugar is "natural" or not.

5 Small Steps to UnDiet

This chapter's Go UnDiet Actions are all about watching out for the little extras that add up to big calories.

▶ **#36. Un-blame carbs and blame the extras instead.** Carbs are not what's making us fat—it's all the stuff we pile on top of them. You don't need to avoid carbs, just limit the extras.

▶ **#37. Un-dip finger foods.** Finger foods are often high-calorie and high-fat to begin with, so avoid adding even more calories and fat by covering them in sauces, dressings, and dips.

▶ **#38. Un-sweeten your drinks.** With an average of 8 teaspoons of sugar in a can of regular soda, it's easy to see how we manage to consume 22 teaspoons of sugar per day. It's okay to add a couple teaspoons of sugar to your coffee, but don't go for drinks with loads of added sugar.

▶ **#39. Un-fake your sugar.** Artificial sweeteners are not a healthy alternative to sugar, and they may even promote weight gain. Instead of faking it with artificial sweeteners, slowly cut back on the amount of sugar you consume.

▶ **#40. Un-source your sugar.** All types of sugar have similar calorie levels and are metabolized by the body in the same way. Natural sugar has no additional nutritional benefits.

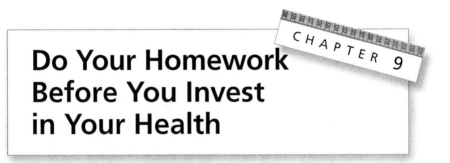

Do Your Homework Before You Invest in Your Health

CHAPTER 9

Investing in your health sounds like a great idea. After all, we invest in our nest eggs, our children, and our homes. Eating functional food—food that promises to boost your health—can seem like killing two birds with one stone. You need to eat anyway, so you may as well eat something that will prevent you from aging or suffering a heart attack. So, how can you tell which food products that promise to boost your health will really deliver on their promises?

Should You Buy Functional Foods?
Can Yogurt Regulate Gut Health and Boost Immunity?
TV commercials claim that yogurt products can prevent constipation, enhance immune functions, or protect your heart. Many yogurt products now carry a claim saying that they can boost gut health or immunity. So, can they really regulate digestive health and prevent you from getting a cold?

The most common bacterial cultures found in yogurt are *L. bulgaricus* and *S. thermophilus*. Dannon's Activia, on the other hand, contains the patented "*bifidus regularis*," which the Dannon website claims will help "regulate your slow intestinal transit." Dannon's yogurt drink, DanActive, claims to help "strengthen your body's defenses" with its trademarked strain "*L. casei immunitas.*" In addition to the usual *L. bulgaricus* and *S. thermophilus*, Yoplait added *Bifodobacterium lactis* to its premium Yo-Plus brand, claiming the extra culture is "clinically shown to support digestive health." Most yogurt products contain active bacterial cultures anyway, so is it worth paying a premium for extra or patented probiotic strains?

Some certainly don't think so. A 2008 class-action lawsuit was launched against Dannon's Activia, accusing the maker of mounting a false advertising campaign to convince consumers to pay more for yogurt. The fact is, not all bacteria strains offer the same health benefits. The most common cultures—*L. bulgaricus* and *S. thermophilus*—are well studied for their ability to reduce symptoms of lactose intolerance and treat diarrhea, particularly in children. The *B. lactis* found in Yo-Plus has been well studied for improving diarrhea and constipation symptoms. The *L. casei* found in DanActive and Yakult has also been well studied for its immune support role. But Dr. Lynne McFarland, Affiliate Associate Professor at the University of Washington, feels that not all yogurt products are well studied. Take the controversial Activia yogurt as an example. "The subjects in the Activia study were not constipated," said McFarland, who is the co-author of *The Power of Probiotics*, a consumer guide to probiotics. "So how does increasing transit time make people healthier?"

Don't allow questionable claims to lead you to write off yogurt, however. It's a nutrition powerhouse—rich in protein and calcium as well as other vitamins and minerals. It can be enjoyed on its own, used as a dip, or mixed into a sauce or dressing.

Go UnDiet Action #41: Un-bank on yogurt to solve constipation.

Yogurt is a dairy food, not a cure for constipation. So don't bank on it to relieve GI distress. The best strategy to relieve constipation is eating lots of fruits and vegetables with enough liquid. Check the yogurt product you have in your fridge and look up its ingredients. Check to see if it contains active bacterial culture (some actually don't!) and make sure it lists the bacterial strains you are looking for. If you use yogurt as an immune-booster, choose one with *L. casei*.

Resource Alert: Use our Go UnDiet Review Tool to compare popular yogurts. http://www.healthcastle.com/product-listing.shtml?catid=5

Can Breakfast Cereals Lower Cholesterol?

Breakfast cereal is a busy person's favorite. It is easy to prepare, and has a satisfying crunch. Plus, it sounds healthy. The most common health claim on cereal boxes is heart-related. Cheerios' website[73] says that Cheerios "can help lower cholesterol and reduce the risk of heart disease". Kellogg's Smart Start Strong Heart cereal and Kashi's Heart To Heart cereal are named in a way that makes it pretty obvious what they intend to suggest.

So, does eating one of these cereals lower your cholesterol levels? Yes, it can—but only if you eat it as not only breakfast, but also lunch, and dinner. Studies show that in people with high cholesterol (above 220 mg/dl), consuming three grams of soluble fiber per day typically lowers total cholesterol by 8–23 percent. One serving of Cheerios (one cup) provides only one gram of soluble fiber, as does Heart To Heart. Are you able to eat three servings of cereals a day?

Before you get desperate, there is good news! There's an often un-promoted ingredient in cereals that may actually lower your cholesterol levels: psyllium. Psyllium does not sound that exciting, especially when you learn that it is the main ingredient in Metamucil. But psyllium in foods is usually found in high concentrations, which means that one serving may contain enough fiber to reach the cholesterol-reducing threshold. Psyllium-containing Kellogg's All Bran Bran Buds cereal, for instance, provides three grams of soluble fiber in just ⅓ cup! Nature's Path's Organic SmartBran also provides three grams of soluble fiber in just one serving thanks to its psyllium content. It's definitely easier to eat one serving of psyllium-containing cereal a day to help lower cholesterol!

 Go UnDiet Action #42: Un-complicate your breakfast cereal.

Don't feel that you should only eat one kind of breakfast cereal. Stock a basic whole grain breakfast cereal as filler and mix it with others you love. For your basic whole grain cereal, choose one that lists whole grain flour as the first ingredient and contains less than four grams of sugar and at least five grams of fiber per serving. To find a cereal that will help lower cholesterol, look for at least three grams of soluble fiber per serving, or look for psyllium seed husk on the ingredient list.

Resource Alert: Use our Go UnDiet Review Tool to compare popular breakfast cereals. http://www.healthcastle. com/product-listing.shtml?catid=1

Can Bread Spread Lower Cholesterol?

Margarine-style spreads that claim to lower cholesterol—like Benecol or Promise Activ—contain plant sterols, which are naturally found in fruit and vegetables in small quantities. The FDA allows products with at least 1.3 grams of plant sterol esters to carry a heart-health claim for reduced coronary heart disease risk. One serving (one tablespoon) of Benecol contains 0.85 grams of plant sterol esters. So, yes—theoretically—two servings of Benecol spread a day can lower cholesterol levels. But before spreading it on your toast two times a day, check out its ingredients.[74]

Benecol—Regular Spread

INGREDIENTS: LIQUID CANOLA OIL, WATER, **PARTIALLY HYDROGENATED SOYBEAN** OIL, PLANT STANOL ESTERS, SALT, EMULSIFIERS, (VEGETABLE MONO- AND DIGLYCERIDES, SOY LECITHIN), HYDROGENATED SOYBEAN OIL, POTASSIUM SORBATE, CITRIC ACID AND CALCIUM DISODIUM EDTA TO PRESERVE FRESHNESS, ARTIFICIAL FLAVOR, DL-ALPHA-TOCOPHERYL ACETATE, VITAMIN A PALMITATE, COLORED WITH BETA CAROTENE.

With chemicals, artificial flavor, emulsifiers, and partially hydrogenated oil, I'm not sure I would eat this two times a day.

Resource Alert: Use our Go UnDiet Review Tool to compare popular spreads. http://www.healthcastle.com/product-listing.shtml?catid=8

> **Verdict:** Plant stenols in other foods may be a better option. Use foods, like whole grains, fresh produce, or cereals with psyllium, to lower cholesterol instead of using plant-sterol bread spread.

Can Exotic Fruit Juice Prevent Aging?

At any given time, there is always an exotic fruit juice making the news. First it was noni juice; more recently it has been pomegranate, mangosteen, acai berry, maqui, and more. Promoters or resellers often boast that their products provide superior levels of antioxidants and can help you fight wrinkles, lose weight, detoxify, or boost energy levels.

Regardless of which juice contains the highest level of antioxidants, there are no scientific studies that show these exotic juices have any extra special health benefits for us.

> **Verdict: Try them if you like their taste and don't need to watch your food budget.** Otherwise, skip the premium juices and spend your hard-earned money on lower-cost antioxidant-rich foods, like fresh produce.

Can Omega 3-Fortified Foods Protect Your Heart?

In Chapter 3, we learned that omega-3s are good fats that are now added to many foods. Omega-3 claims can be found on many food products, including orange juice, snack bars, breakfast cereals, and milk and yogurt. But do these foods have the right kind of omega-3?

Let's take Quaker Fiber & Omega-3 Chewy Oat Granola Bars as an example. The box says the snack bar is an "excellent source of fiber and omega-3." Reading the ingredient list, we learn that it contains plant-based ALA from flaxseeds. In Chapter 3, we discussed plant-based omega-3 (ALA) and marine-based omega-3 (EPA & DHA). We know that marine-based EPA & DHA, but not plant-based ALA, are effective in lowering LDL cholesterol and triglyceride levels. So how does eating a snack bar with ALA help protect our health?

What about omega-3 enriched eggs? Chicken farmers use special feeds so their chicken will produce eggs enriched with omega-3. Most of these eggs are from chicken fed with a flaxseed diet. Aha! Flaxseed—that's plant-based ALA again! They don't do much to protect your heart. Some farmers, on the other hand, add fish oil to chicken feed to boost DHA in eggs. So look for eggs that clearly show their DHA levels on the carton. Most brands of these DHA eggs have 100–150 mg of DHA per egg.

So, the key is to look for DHA on the label. But be careful: Even if you find this term on the label, you may be disappointed with what you find on the Nutrition Facts panel. Take Horizon Organic DHA Omega-3 milk as an example. It clearly includes DHA in its product name, but its level is surprisingly low at 32 mg of DHA per serving. The recommended daily level is 500 mg of DHA + EPA. So, to answer the question, do omega-3 enriched foods protect your heart? Yes—theoretically—but you will have to eat a lot of these DHA-enriched foods to reach the recommended level!

Verdict: Don't bank on DHA-enriched foods to lower your cholesterol levels—they should be viewed only as supplementary. **Eat fish instead.** A three-ounce serving of salmon has 1,000 to 1,500 mg of DHA + EPA! Just two servings of fish a week will meet your needs.

What About Soy?

Among all the health food claims, soy has gotten to be the most confusing. Soy was crowned by the FDA in October 1999 and was approved for labeling foods containing soy protein as protective against heart disease. But in 2007, The U.S. Agency for Healthcare Research and Quality analyzed various soy studies. They found that soy only had a modest effect on cholesterol levels. They found that eating a high amount of soy protein only caused a 3% reduction in LDL cholesterol levels, not as impressive as once claimed. This prompted the American Heart Association Nutrition Committee to issue an advisory in January 2006,[75] rescinding its position to recommend soy foods to lower cholesterol.

One of the main reasons there was such a fiasco is that soy products vary. The kind of soy products I'm familiar with are made with a set of pestle & mortar, a cheese cloth, plus whole soybeans. This was the way my vegetarian grandma made soy milk and tofu! One cup of cooked soybeans has 7.6 grams of fiber, and a nutrient profile of approximately ⅓ distribution each of carb, protein, and fat. But if you look carefully at the label of soy products available now, you will find ingredients like "soy protein isolates," "soy protein concentrates," and "textured vegetable (or soy) protein." These are very different from whole soybeans! Isolates are mostly protein and have only 3% carb content. They hardly have any fat or fiber left. Soy protein concentrates, on the other hand, contain about 70% protein and 20% carb. They also have almost no fat, but retain more fiber than soy protein isolates. The process of dehulling, defattening, and flaking soybeans virtually remove isoflavones—the potential beneficial components found in soy. According to a 2004 scientific review,[76] soy flour retains 50% more isoflavones than defatted soybean flakes. Soy protein concentrates extracted by alcohol, however, retain only 6% of the isoflavones that soy flour can.

I don't mean to confuse you by listing all these soy ingredients, but that's the reality. Some packaged foods are over-processed, and so are some soy ingredients. Whether soy can lower cholesterol remains to be studied. With its high content of PUFA (poly-unsaturated fatty acids), fiber, and nutrients, soy certainly is a healthy food, especially when it is used to replace animal meat.

 Go UnDiet Action #43: Un-soy-erize.
Don't get me wrong—soy is good. But stick to natural soy products—like tofu, soy nuts, soy butter, edamame, and some soy milk, and stay away from highly processed soy products like soy snack bars, chicken-tasting soy meat, soy patties or sausages, soy whipped cream, and soy cream.

Does Vitamin Water Keep You Healthy?

Tasteless plain water is not very exciting. On the other hand, colorful, sweet, enhanced water—water with vitamins and flavors added—is more fun and sexy. But can it "help keep you healthy as a horse," as claimed on the label of Coca-Cola-owned Glaceau's Defense Vitaminwater?

Most brands of enhanced water have some B vitamins added, such as B3, B6, and B12. Some may add Vitamins C or E, or zinc. Dasani Plus Refresh + Revive enhanced water, for instance, has 10% of the recommended daily intake of Vitamins B3, B6 and B12 per serving. According to CDC's National Health and Nutrition Examination Survey (NHANES),[77] we already consume *more than* the recommended levels on all three B vitamins. So how does the

extra 10% from Dasani Plus help us refresh and revive? And is
it worth paying $1.50 for a bottle of water to get these vitamins?

You may argue that that $1.50 also buys you palate stimuli (i.e.,
sweetness) and visual stimuli (i.e., coloring). But what's the real
cost? The calorie content ranges from 0 to 130 calories per bottle,
with varying levels of artificial sweeteners and sugar. At 0 calories,
Skinny Water contains two artificial sweeteners. At 130 calories,
8 teaspoons of sugar are added to Glaceau's Vitaminwater.

Product	Flavor	Bottle Size	Calories Per Bottle	Sweetening Agents
Plain water	Plain		0	None
Skinny Water (Total-V)	Lemonade Passion Fruit	16 oz.	0	Acesulfame potassium, sucralose
SoBe 0 Cal Lifewater	Yumberry Pomegranate	20 oz.	10	Erythritol, Reb A
Propel	Kiwi Strawberry	20 oz.	25	Sugar, sucralose, acesulfame potassium
SoBe Lifewater	Strawberry Kiwi	20 oz.	100	Sugar, erythritol
Snapple Antioxidant Water	Strawberry Acai	20 oz.	125	Sugar
Vitaminwater— Defense	Raspberry-Apple	20 oz.	130	Cane sugar

Table 22. Sweetening agents in some common enhanced waters

Don't expect to find real fruit juice in these enhanced waters,
either. Neither strawberry nor kiwi ingredients were found in SoBe's
Lifewater Strawberry Kiwi. Instead, you will find sweet potato
juice as a coloring agent.

> **Verdict: Don't expect enhanced water to enhance your health.** It may be a better alternative than soda. However, if you absolutely crave pink water, you can make a much healthier version by freezing some cut-up red fruit, such as strawberries, overnight and using them as ice cubes in plain water.

Should You Take Supplements?

According to the National Institutes of Health, at least half of American adults take a supplement. People often treat supplements as health insurance—it's kind of like a top-up to cover the gaps. Use the following do-it-yourself assessment to find out if you need any supplements. **Caution:** The following assessment does not apply to people with chronic medical conditions. Always check with your physicians before taking any supplements.

Do-It-Yourself: 6 Questions to Ask Yourself Before Taking Any Supplements

1. Do you smoke?
2. Do you wear sunscreen all the time?
3. Are you over 50?
4. Are you pregnant, or do you plan to get pregnant?
5. Are you eating less than three daily servings of dairy or other calcium-rich foods?
6. Are you eating less than two weekly servings of fish?

If you answered "Yes" to any of the above questions, you may want to consider taking a supplement. Let's get into the details on each of the questions above:

1. Smoking is probably the single greatest cause of preventable medical conditions. Smoking causes damage to the body that even the healthiest eating habits cannot help. So, if quitting is not an option, it is a good idea to take daily basic multivitamins. But make sure to choose one that does not exceed 100% of the DV (daily value) for any vitamins. In particular, choose one with low or no beta-carotene. Studies have found that beta-carotene supplementation actually increases lung cancer rates among smokers and cardiovascular disease rates among female smokers.

2. If you wear sunscreen all year round, your skin is not able to produce Vitamin D from direct sunlight, so you may want to consider taking Vitamin D supplements. Vitamin D is also found in dairy, fatty fish, and egg yolks, but the amount is low. Studies have shown multiple benefits of Vitamin D, including prevention of cancer and osteoporosis. Indeed, in Canada, routine daily Vitamin D supplementation of 1,000 IU is recommended for all adults during the winter months as a cancer-preventative measure.

3. Lower stomach acid production as we age reduces our ability to absorb Vitamin B12 from food. If you also take acid reflux medication, you may have even less acid. Also, as body functions change, our needs for Vitamins B6, D, and calcium actually increase with age. Increased nutrient needs can usually be achieved by eating more foods. But for people over 50, calorie needs actually decrease as activity level usually decreases and metabolism slows, and hence less food is eaten. Because of the changes, a daily multivitamin may be needed for people over 50.

4. If you are pregnant, you are probably already taking a daily multivitamin and mineral supplement. If you are planning

to conceive in the near future, you should start taking a folic acid supplement of at least 400 micrograms (or 0.4 mg). Folic acid is crucial in neonatal neural tube formation—occurring in the first trimester of pregnancy. Babies with folic acid deficiency may be born with neural tube defects—when the neural tube fails to close during the early stages of pregnancy, which may result in physical and developmental disabilities such as spina bifida. Sometimes, women don't know they are pregnant until they've missed their monthly menstrual cycle. By that time, they can already be three to four weeks pregnant. Therefore, taking a folic acid supplement in the planning stage before a pregnancy is crucial.

5. The recommended daily calcium requirement for both women and men between the ages of 19 and 50 is 1,000 mg, and for men over 50 it's 1,200 mg. One serving of dairy or other calcium-fortified drink like orange juice or soymilk provides about 290 mg—so most women need at least three servings to meet the requirement. If you are not eating or drinking many high-calcium foods, consider taking a calcium supplement.

Go UnDiet Action #44: Be un-swayed by fancy calcium marketing.

Don't be confused by the fancy marketing when shopping for calcium supplements. Look for the content of "elemental calcium" only. Calcium supplements are available in numerous forms: pills, capsules, enteric-coated pills, powder, liquid, or chewable. They may be synthetic, "natural from plant sources," "naturally occurring from oyster shell," or "natural from coral bed." In addition, they may be acidic, alkaline or neutral in pH. They may also be bundled with Vitamin D, magnesium, Vitamin K, glucosamine sulphate or more. No wonder we are confused! Just remember one thing—the reason you are buying calcium supplements is because you want to supplement your diet with calcium. It is good to have other nutrients, especially Vitamin D, that aid calcium absorption, but there is only so much that pill manufacturers can jam into one pill. Too many extra ingredients often reduce the amount of elemental calcium present in the pill (which means you have to take more pills a day to cover your calcium needs), or render it too big to swallow. So choose one mainly based on the amount of elemental calcium you need.

6. We've discussed fish multiple times in this book already, so by now you should know the health benefits of marine-based omega-3—DHA and EPA. If you eat fish less than two times a week and have no plans to increase fish intake, consider taking a fish oil supplement. If you are a vegetarian, you can take algae oil DHA supplements.

If you decide to take a multivitamin (or your doctor recommends that you do), beware of high-potency formulations. The strongest formula is not always the best choice. Too much of certain vitamins and minerals such as Vitamin A or iron in your multivitamin supplement can actually be harmful. Let me explain why.

Three Micronutrients You Shouldn't Take Too Much Of
Vitamin A: The recommended level of Vitamin A is 3,000 IU daily for adult men and 2,310 IU for women. Some multivitamins have 10,000 IU packed into a daily dose. Too much Vitamin A can lead to birth defects, liver abnormalities, reduced bone mineral density (which may in turn result in osteoporosis), and central nervous

system disorders. As a general rule, look for a multivitamin that contains no more than 4,000 IU of Vitamin A.

Vitamin E: The recommended level of Vitamin E is 22.5 IU daily for both men and women. But some multivitamins are packed with 400–800 IU of Vitamin E. This is particularly dangerous because a daily dose of 400 IU or more of Vitamin E can increase the risk of death from all causes, according to a 2005 Vitamin E study[78] conducted by Johns Hopkins University. Furthermore, a head and neck cancer study[79] found that cancer patients receiving a daily dose of 400 IU of Vitamin E during and after radiation therapy were at *greater* risk of developing a second primary cancer. Although the findings are still inconclusive, the highly regarded Center of Science in the Public Interest (CSPI) recommends choosing a multivitamin that contains no more than 100 IU of Vitamin E.

Iron: The recommended level of iron is 8 mg daily for men, 18 mg for premenopausal women, and 8 mg for menopausal women. Too much iron can cause constipation. In addition, studies in the 1980s reported that high iron stores in men were associated with high risk of heart attacks. CSPI recommends choosing a multivitamin that contains no more than 10 mg of iron for men and postmenopausal women, and 14–18 mg for premenopausal women.

Go UnDiet Action #45: Un-generalize your multis. If you are recommended (or decide) to take a multivitamin supplement, choose one that does not contain over 100 percent of the DV of any vitamins. Also, choose one that is gender-specific and age-specific. That's because our needs vary by gender and age. For instance, men need a lot less iron than women, and too much iron is actually harmful for men. Women over 50 need less iron, but more calcium and Vitamins D and B12 than women under 50.

UnDiet Q&A: Do you need a multivitamin if you don't eat enough fruit and vegetables?

Every time I talk about supplements, this question is always raised. If you are not eating enough fruit and vegetables, you should increase your intake of fruit and vegetables, not pop a pill. This may not be what you want to hear. But if you are not eating enough fruit and veggies, chances are you are overeating other foods. We all need to eat a certain volume of food to feel full, so if you are not eating enough low-calorie-density fruit and vegetables, you are very likely filling up your stomach by eating more meat, grains, or snacks, which are higher-calorie-dense. Popping a pill may help you fill the gaps of the missing nutrients, but it does not make you feel full. Studies[80,81] have shown that simply increasing your fruit and vegetable intake can help you lose weight significantly faster than just trying to cut down on high-fat or high-sugar foods.

5 Small Steps to UnDiet

This chapter's Go UnDiet Actions are all about health claims on food and supplements. Not all health claims are worth investing in.

▶ **#41. Un-bank on yogurt to solve constipation.** Eat your yogurt as a dairy food, not a constipation relief.

▶ **#42. Un-complicate your breakfast cereal.** Stock a basic whole grain breakfast cereal as filler and mix it with others you love. Choose one that lists whole grain flour as the first ingredient and contains less than four grams of sugar and at least five grams of fiber per serving.

▶ **#43. Un-soy-erize.** Eat natural soy foods, not fancy soy snacks made with partial soy ingredients.

▶ **#44. Be un-swayed by fancy calcium marketing.** Focus on elemental calcium content when choosing a calcium supplement, not the extras.

▶ **#45. Un-generalize your multis.** Choose a multivitamin supplement that is gender-specific and age-specific.

CHAPTER 10

Look Beyond Calories

Now that you've read through 45 Go UnDiet Action steps and tried many of them, it's time to learn some new skills and behaviors that will help you stick to your action goals.

The Weakest Link

In the previous chapters, you've learned how to spot highly processed foods, or HPF. Many HPF are empty-calorie foods—a fancy new term for what we used to just call "junk food." And empty-calorie foods are indeed the weakest link when it comes to establishing healthy eating patterns and reaching your weight-loss goals.

What are Empty-Calorie Foods?

What are empty-calorie foods, and why are they so bad for you? The definition is simple: Empty-calorie foods are high in sugar, fat, and/or calories, and low in nutrition. That is, they don't have a lot of vitamins or minerals. Take a look at Table 23 for some examples of empty-calorie foods.

Food category	Examples	Why to Avoid
Deep-fried foods	• french fries • chips	A large order of fries from a fast-food chain can contain up to 570 calories with a whopping 30 g of total fat and 8 g of trans fat! Tons of calories from fat and very few nutrients.
Sweetened packaged foods	• candy • soda and other sweetened drinks	A can of soda contains about 130 calories as well as additives and colorings. Again, lots of calories from sugar but no nutrients.
Alcoholic beverages	• beer • coolers	A can of beer contains about 150 calories from sugar and not much of anything else. In addition, calories from alcohol tend to be stored as fat in the abdomen (leading to a "beer belly").
Refined grains	• crackers • cookies	Refined grains do provide some B vitamins, but that's it.

Table 23. Empty-calorie foods

Now that you know how to spot empty-calorie foods, and understand why you should avoid them, you won't be easily swayed by sneaky marketing that tries to convince you junk foods can actually be good for you. So when you see candy bars that claim to have beneficial phytonutrients, exotic juices that claim to help you lose weight, sugary water that claims to boost your energy or your immune system, potato chips that claim to be good for the earth, or corn chips that say they "contain the goodness of whole grain," think back to this chapter and remember that empty calories are always empty calories, even if the product packaging makes impressive health claims.

Go UnDiet Action #46: Un-empty your calories.
No matter how the product packaging claims it's good for you or the earth, junk foods are just junk foods, and adding a few nutrients back in doesn't make them health foods.

Eat at the Table
Where You Eat is as Important as What You Eat

We used to eat at one place: the table. But somehow, over the past 20 years, we've moved from eating in the kitchen or the dining room to anyplace where our hands are free, like in front of the TV, at the computer, at the football game, or even in the car—when our hands really shouldn't be free for eating at all!

This transition to eating on the run has also marked a change in the kinds of foods we eat—since you're not likely to cook a well-balanced meal and then eat it while you drive. People who eat on the run end up eating whatever food is easily and quickly available, so they have higher intakes of soda, fast food, total fat, and saturated fat. Women who eat on the run have also been found to have lower intakes of fruit, vegetables, and fiber.[82]

There are many reasons why you should consider eating to be an activity in itself, rather than something to do to keep your hands busy, or something you can get out of the way while focusing on something else. Mindful eating—paying attention to what you are eating, rather than just cramming food into your mouth—helps you listen to your body and make conscious eating decisions. It allows you to slow the pace of your eating, so you can learn to recognize your body's hunger cues, and eat only when you're hungry and stop when you're full.

Mindful eating can have a huge impact on your weight-loss goals. In fact, research shows that practicing mindful eating is actually more effective for weight loss than following a rigid diet plan.[83] Your body really is programmed to help you achieve a healthy weight—if you're willing to listen to what it tells you.

 Go UnDiet Action #47: Un-dashboard dine.
Make dining a priority and schedule it into your day, just like you schedule your other activities. Stop mindless eating and eating in front of the TV or computer. This will help you learn to recognize your body's signals and stop overeating, or eating when you're not hungry.

Get Cooking!

Throughout the book, I've been discouraging you from snacking on HPF. They are easy temptations—they are so easy to overeat. Just open the bag. That's it! They are not fresh, and some of them are not even food!

I always advocate home cooking. Home cooking guarantees you and your family are eating real food. To find out your daily amount of foods from each food group based on your calorie needs, refer to Appendix B in this book.

It Doesn't Have to be Complicated

Let's face it. Do you spend more time fixing your hair and makeup than fixing meals? If you are willing to spend an hour every morning fixing yourself, but protest that preparing for dinner takes too much time, you're probably just not ready to cook. And that's okay. Everyone has different priorities.

But if healthy eating is high on your priority list, then home-cooked meals are always the best option. The best meal is always a meal that is prepared by you. I trust foods that are made by humans much more than foods that are made by machines. So, that means that learning to put together a meal is a basic skill for healthy eating.

Cooking is a learning process, and what you create does not need to be gourmet to achieve your eating goals. When I was a teenager, I used to be very proud of my creamy pasta creation, which involved a sauce made from Campbell's cream of mushroom soup. That was the best I could come up with! My younger sister Janette, on the other hand, was a chef from the start. Every Saturday morning, she would spend 30–45 minutes creating a breakfast of traditional steel-cut oatmeal with egg wash and just the right amount of milk—and she was only 14! My point is that we all need to start somewhere, and just because you don't think you're as good a cook as other people you know (or the people you see on TV), that doesn't mean you shouldn't try to create healthy meals at home.

We all need to start from whatever level we're at, then add skills as we go. You wouldn't laugh at a child learning to swim with a flotation device, so you certainly don't need to feel ashamed about using some "aids" to help you as you learn to cook. My cream of mushroom pasta didn't offer a whole lot of nutritional value, but it was still better than a meal at a fast-food restaurant. And it got me used to spending time in the kitchen, so when I was ready to start moving on to more serious cooking, at least I knew where everything was and how to work the stove!

My point is that you can start at whatever level you feel comfortable with. Making a vegetable soup with a low-sodium canned stock as the base is a great example. It's much easier than creating your soup stock from scratch, and you end up with a healthy meal with lots of vegetables. The key is to start the process, because once you've started home cooking, you will start advancing and want to try even new recipes more.

Make the Foods You Love

The best way to learn how to cook is to start making foods you love by following the recipe. Start with just one favorite dish. Once you are comfortable with that recipe, look for information on different ways to cook the same main ingredient, like roasting, stir-frying, steaming, braising, and so on. Learning various cooking techniques is important—this will create variety (and less waste) in your cooking. Even if you make chicken three nights in a row, your dishes can be completely different if you use different cooking methods to prepare them.

If you feel like you need some step-by-step directions, there are many resources available to you without enrolling in a professional culinary school. Check out your local community center or college—many of them offer basic cooking classes. It was a local college cooking course that taught me the first skills I needed to move beyond mushroom soup sauce!

You can also check out online videos. There's even an online cooking school that's dedicated to teaching basic techniques (rather than specific fancy recipes) through numerous video cooking classes. You can find it at Rouxbe.com.

You can also check out the No More Packaged Foods series of recipes on my website at http://www.healthcastle.com/nomore_packaged_foods_home.shtml. It explains how to create homemade versions of favorite foods like pasta sauce or fish sticks with basic ingredients, usually in only slightly more time than it takes to heat up the boxed version.

Go UnDiet Action #48: Un-shun cooking.
Home cooking is more than just boiling pasta and heating up jarred pasta sauce. Start with the basics and develop your skills as you go.

Get Your Family Involved

As I've emphasized many times throughout this book, it's important to make healthy eating a family priority. And because it should be a priority for the whole family, every family member should contribute to the cooking effort. Try taking a cooking class with your spouse, or getting your teenaged kids to take responsibility for one or two meals a week. Or, you could all cook together as a family, with each person taking responsibility for a certain task, or a certain part of the meal. You can even get young kids involved by showing them how to make simple dishes, and getting them to help out with tasks that don't involve sharp knives or hot pans. You'll be surprised by how much the little things your family does can help.

If you're pressed for time, you can also look into using a grocery delivery service or joining a CSA (as discussed in Chapter 7). The key is to make healthy eating as easy as possible!

Go UnDiet Action #49: Un-burden yourself.
Make healthy eating easy. Get help from your family with cooking and grocery shopping, or have your food

delivered by a grocery delivery service or CSA. (You can find a list of CSAs at http://www.localharvest.org/CSA.)

Stop Counting Calories

I've given this last section—and the Go UnDiet Action that goes with it—a lot of thought. Every time I speak about nutrition in public, someone always approaches me to ask if they should switch to skim milk or fat-free yogurt, or if they should switch from one cooking oil to another. You know how I feel about fat-free products (I think I made my point pretty clearly in Chapter 2!), so I won't repeat myself. But I've always been puzzled by these questions—since they tend to be so similar, and always focus on identifying one option as "good" and the other as "bad." I think the people who ask me if they should switch to, say, olive oil, want me to tell them that olive oil is "good." But even if it's good, that doesn't mean you can feel better about using lots of it in your cooking! All of this has led me to come to a conclusion—some of us are obsessed with rigid rules and "bad" foods.

I've mentioned some of the rules people set for themselves in other chapters, like eating 3 meals plus 1 snack, or eating foods with more than five ingredients. These rules may come from good intentions, but they can become an obsession. It's human nature to want to break the rules—anything that's forbidden is automatically more exciting. Inevitably, when you set rigid rules for yourself, you end up breaking them. And since you're breaking the rules anyway, you tend to have a lot of your "bad" food instead of just a little. Then you just feel guilty, and you try to make yourself feel better by telling yourself that the "bad" food you ate that broke the rules was an indulgence or decadence. But that just makes the foods that break your rules even more appealing, and it makes you even more likely to gravitate toward these indulgent, decadent foods when you are stressed or upset.

Do you see it now? This kind of negotiating with yourself over rigid rules is a vicious cycle that doesn't end.

And calories are only one aspect of food. Snacking on low-calorie foods does not always mean that you are eating fewer overall calories. Research[84] has shown that eating low-fat foods leads to a decrease in fat, but not overall calorie intake. In other words, low-fat products do not help you reduce overall calorie intake. That's probably because people over-compensate, either eating more of the low-fat foods, or eating more foods in subsequent meals thereafter.

Go UnDiet Action #50: Un-count calories.
Eating healthy is not about choosing the food with the lowest calories possible. Don't get obsessed with calories and "bad" foods. Instead, create a healthy eating atmosphere by making eating a happy occasion—a sit-down family time to prepare food together and socialize. Plainly put, almost anything you create in your own kitchen will be healthier (and have fewer calories) than fat-laden fast food items and additive-laden HPF.

5 Small Steps to UnDiet

This chapter ties the actions you've tried in the rest of the book together, and teaches you some basic skills and behaviors you'll need to keep your UnDiet going once you get to the final pages of this book.

- ▶ **#46. Un-empty your calories.** Junk foods are just that—junk foods. Despite some marketing promises, adding in a few nutrients does not make them good for you.

- ▶ **#47. Un-dashboard dine.** Make time to pay attention to what you're eating. Mindful eating is an important factor in achieving your weight-loss goals.

- ▶ **#48. Un-shun cooking.** A little bit of home cooking is better than none, and you don't have to be a gourmet chef to enjoy the benefits. Start with short, easy recipes and work your way up from there.

- ▶ **#49. Unburden yourself.** Get help with shopping and cooking. You can even get your groceries delivered!

- ▶ **#50. Un-count calories.** Eating healthy is not all about counting calories or grams of fat. The steps in this book have taught you how to make healthy choices without obsessing about numbers and rules.

CHAPTER 11

Putting It All Together

You've learned a lot of things in this book. But if there is one lesson that I want you to take away from all of the reading, all of the small changes, and all of the Go UnDiet Actions, it's this: Life is about choices. You face a series of choices every single day, starting the very moment you wake up—what time to get out of bed, what clothes to wear, how you get to work, who you talk to, and how you spend your time. And, of course, every day you make choices about what you eat.

You Are in the Driver's Seat

We are facing an obesity epidemic. It's easy to point the finger for this problem at the government, food manufacturers, fast food giants, and restaurants, but the fact is that only you can decide what you put into your mouth. No matter how good something tastes, or how much advertising you have watched to persuade you to buy a certain food product or go to a restaurant chain, nothing gets into your body without you making the decision to take it in.

Only you can change your diet, and ultimately your health. But it can be hard to know where to start. This book has helped you put your own diet under a microscope and break it into smaller pieces so you can work on it in manageable stages, piece by piece.

Now that you have worked through all of the UnDiet Actions, you should be in control of your own food choices. But it may be hard to remember some of the actions you took in the beginning. It's a good idea to take a quick look back at the Go UnDiet Actions at the end of each chapter as a refresher from time to time. But here's a simple summary to guide you in your day-to-day food choices.

Eat More...
Fiber

As you learned in Chapter 4, surveys show we only eat half as much fiber as we need. This is a big deal. Why? Because fiber is essential for a healthy body, plus it helps reduce the risk for several chronic diseases, and even some cancers. It can even help lower your bad LDL cholesterol and help manage diabetes by lowering blood sugar.

Take a look back at Go UnDiet Actions 16, 17, 18 and 20 in Chapter 4:

- **Go UnDiet Action 16.** Un-favor whole grain logos: Most whole grain logos are not a guarantee of good whole grain content.

- **Go UnDiet Action 17.** Uncover whole: Look for the word "whole" on labels to indicate whole grains.

- **Go UnDiet Action 18.** Unleash whole grains from breakfast: Try serving whole grains at lunch or dinner.

- ![Go UnDiet icon] **Go UnDiet Action 20.** Un-halt your grains; let them sprout. Try sprouted grains for a softer texture.

Potassium

Potassium can actually help to counter the effect of too much sodium by allowing your kidneys to excrete the excess. As you learned in Chapter 2, we tend to get far more sodium than we should. Potassium can help (though don't think you have an excuse to load up on sodium every time you eat potassium-rich foods!). Potassium can be found in bananas, beans, tofu, and potatoes, as well as many fruits and vegetables. You can find a good list of potassium-rich foods in Table 2.

Vitamin D

As you learned in Chapter 9, some of us are not getting enough of all the vitamins and minerals we need to stay healthy, and if you wear sunscreen every day or are over 50, getting more Vitamin D is especially important. Vitamin D has been shown to have many benefits, including preventing cancer and osteoporosis. It also aids calcium absorption.

Vitamin D is found in small amounts in dairy, fatty fish, and egg yolks, but only in small amounts, so you may need to add a Vitamin D supplement to your daily routine.

Whole Ingredients

Remember my story from Chapter 10 about cooking pasta with a mushroom soup sauce as a teenager? I've come a long way since then, and you will too, once you start cooking at home and discovering your favorite ingredients. Foods made by humans are much more nutritious than the HPF made by machines, and cooking at home gives you a new way to interact with your family, as well. Start with the foods you love, and learn techniques from online sources like Rouxbe.com. You can also find some easy recipes on my website at http://www.healthcastle.com/nomore_packaged_foods_home.shtml.

Take a look back at Go UnDiet Action 48 in Chapter 10:

- **Go UnDiet Action 48.** Un-shun cooking: Move beyond heating up packaged food. Start simple and learn as you go.

We've compiled a list of Top 60 Super Foods in Appendix D. These foods were compiled based on the above recommendations— eat more fiber, potassium, Vitamin D, and whole ingredients.

And Eat Less...

It all comes down to what I talked about in Chapter 2: The biggest culprit for our weight problems is overeating on the worst offenders! We snack when we're not hungry, and we snack on the worst-offending HPF!

So, we should cut out or eat less:

Added Sugar from Liquid Calories

As I explained in Chapters 6 and 8, drinking calories is the number one reason why we are overweight. We drink between 450 and 550 calories per day—and 60% of those calories are from sweetened drinks like soda, bottled iced tea, sports drinks, chocolate milk, and so on. To make it worse, researchers have found a link between drinking sugar-sweetened drinks and weight gain in both adults and children. Our bodies need water, not sugar-laden drinks!

Take a look back at Go UnDiet Actions 26 and 28 in Chapter 6, and Action 38 in Chapter 8:

- **Go UnDiet Action 26.** Un-drink your calories: Your drinks should be a source of water for your body, not unnecessary calories that don't make you feel full.

- **Go UnDiet Action 28:** Understand the UnDiet formula: 3+1. If needed, drink only one sweetened drink a day.

- **Go UnDiet Action 38.** Un-sweeten your drinks: Avoid soda and other sweetened drinks. They are packed with sugar.

Sodium from HPF

As you saw in Chapter 2, we currently eat about 50% more sodium than we should, and much of that extra sodium comes from highly processed foods like soup, frozen dinners, instant noodles, processed meats, and so on. That's a big concern for health officials—and for you—because too much sodium can increase your risk of high blood pressure and other heart diseases. Cutting down on HPF is one easy way to cut your intake of sodium.

Take a look back at Go UnDiet Action 6 in Chapter 2:

- **Go UnDiet Action 6:** Un-low: The only "low" claim that's really a good thing is low sodium.

Solid Fats from HPF

We often hear about the saturated fat in meat, and we've been trained to worry about its effects. But you learned in Chapter 3 that solid fats from HPF are a much bigger problem, because we get way more bad saturated fat from HPF than we ever could from healthy cuts of meat.

Take a look back at Go UnDiet Actions 12 and 15 in Chapter 3:

- **Go UnDiet Action 12:** Un-HPF: Stick to food in its most natural form, and avoid HPF as much as possible.

- **Go UnDiet Action 15:** Un-palm: The presence of this solid fat is an indication that the product is likely highly processed.

In other words, cut out the empty calories listed in Chapter 10 and the worst offending HPF suggested in Chapter 2!

The Bottom Line

Don't forget: You should not try to live with a rigid meal plan. You should adopt a total approach that allows you to incorporate your own food preferences and fully participate in social occasions. It's not the end of the world if you overeat at your family Thanksgiving dinner. Really, it's okay—as long as you are mindful of what you're doing and get right back on track. It only becomes an issue if you start coming up with creative excuses to overeat every week. So stop giving yourself excuses for eating poorly and not being happy with the way you look or feel. Take control of your food choices now! It's time to stop dieting, enjoy eating fresh, whole, healthy foods, and Go UnDiet.

For a complete list of all 50 Go UnDiet Actions, refer to Appendix E.

Summary of Nutrition Requirements for an Average Healthy Adult (aged 19–50)

APPENDIX A

Calories
Female: 1,800–2,400 calories per day
Male: 2,200–3,000 calories per day

Fiber
Female: 25 grams per day
Male: 38 grams per day

Carbohydrates
Female: ~ 130 grams per day
Male: ~ 130 grams per day

Protein
Female: ~ 46 grams per day
Male: ~ 56 grams per day

Source: Dietary Reference Intakes for Energy, Carbohydrate, Fiber, Fat, Fatty Acids, Cholesterol, Protein, and Amino Acids (2002).

To find out your exact calorie requirement, use our free Calorie Calculator at http://www.healthcastle.com/calorie-requirement-calculator.shtml.

Amount of Food Required from Each Group Per Day[85]

Calorie level	1,800 kcal	2,000	2,200	2,400	2,600	2,800	3,000 kcal
Meat (oz.)	5	5.5	6	6.5	6.5	7	7
Grains (servings)	6	6	7	8	9	10	10
Veggies (servings)	2.5	2.5	3	3	3.5	3.5	4
Fruits (servings)	1.5	2	2	2	2	2.5	2.5
Milk (cups)	3	3	3	3	3	3	3

30 Snacks under 200 Calories

The best snack option is always fruit or vegetables. Many of them are under 100 calories per serving, and are full of fiber and antioxidants. For the snackers who want more than just fruit or something different, HealthCastle.com contributing writer Beth Ehrensberger, MPH, RD, has put together these 30 snack combos.

	Calories	Fiber
1 lettuce wrap made with a lettuce leaf, 1 ounce chicken meat and one teaspoon mustard	70	0.6
1 cantaloupe wedge and ½ ounce almonds (11 nuts)	105	2.4
1 part-skim mozzarella string cheese stick and 1 cup cherry tomatoes	116	1.6
1 cup unshelled Edamame (sprinkled with sea salt if desired)	130	5.7
2 deviled egg halves and 1 cup celery sticks	133	2.0
1 Asian pear and ½ ounce cashews (about 9 nuts)	134	4.9

½ cup 2% cottage cheese with ½ cup fresh pineapple chunks	136	1.1
10 bite-size pretzels and 1 tablespoon peanut butter	139	1.3
1 ounce reduced-fat provolone cheese slice melted over ½ of a whole grain English muffin	142	2.4
½ of a whole grain waffle topped with ¼ cup low-fat yogurt and 1 small, sliced peach	143	2.5
½ cup oven-roasted garbanzo beans (with sea salt if desired)	148	7.0
1 packet instant oatmeal with 2 tablespoons 2% milk	148	2.6
1 12-oz. coffee shop latte made with 2% milk	150	0.0
1 8-oz. coffee shop hot chocolate made with 2% milk	160	0.0
2 clementines and 2 tablespoons shelled pistachio nuts	161	4.2
1 cup canned, reduced-sodium tomato soup and 4 whole grain crackers	161	3.5
1 cup 1% milk and 1 graham cracker sheet	162	0.4
1 slice of 100% whole wheat bread spread with 1 tablespoon almond butter	165	2.4
½ ounce 70% dark chocolate and 1 cup unpitted cherries	172	4.4
6 oz. plain low-fat yogurt topped with 2 tablespoons granola	175	1.5
1 mini whole wheat bagel with a scrambled egg topped with one tablespoon salsa	175	2.8
½ cup carrot sticks, 3 tablespoons hummus, 4 inch whole wheat pita	181	5.0
3 tablespoons roasted sunflower seed kernels and ½ cup raspberries	182	6.7

1 cup whole grain cereal, ½ cup 1% milk, ¼ cup blueberries	182	4.0
¾ cup 2% chocolate milk and 10 strawberries	185	3.7
¼ cup guacamole, 4 whole grain crackers, ½ cup red pepper sticks	186	6.9
½ ounce walnuts (7 halves), 2 tablespoons dried cranberries, ¼ cup whole grain cereal	188	3.0
½ cup grapes, ½ ounce chunk parmesan cheese, 4 low-sodium whole grain crackers	188	2.8
2 cups air-popped popcorn tossed with a tablespoon olive oil and a teaspoon each of chilli and garlic powder.	199	3.5
1 small pear, 1 ounce sharp cheddar cheese	200	4.6

Top 60 Super Foods

Almonds	Bok choy	Eggplant
Amaranth	Broccoli	Figs
Apricot	Brown rice	Flax seeds
Asparagus	Bulgur	Green tea
Avocado	Cherries, any	Hazelnuts
Banana	Chia seeds	Hemp seeds
Barley	Chickpeas	Kale
Beans & lentils, any	Coffee	Kiwi
Beets	Concord grapes	Milk, organic
Bitter melon	Dark chocolate	Millet
Black rice	Dried plums	Mushrooms, any
Blueberries	Edamame	Oats

Peanuts	Sorghum	Sweet potato
Pecans	Soy nuts	Tofu
Pistachios	Spinach	Tomato
Pumpkin	Squash, any	Walnuts
Pumpkin seeds	Strawberries	Whole rye
Quinoa	Sunflower seeds	Wild rice
Salmon	Swiss chard	Yogurt

Many readers often ask, "Which super foods should I eat more of?" I hear this question a lot! Indeed, the Super Foods section of my website (http://www.healthcastle.com/food_supplements.shtml) is among the top 3 most popular sections.

The list compiled above is based on my recommendation in Chapter 11 to eat more

- Fiber

- Potassium

- Vitamin D, and

- Whole ingredients

50 Small Actions to UnDiet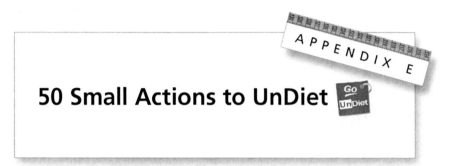

☐ **#1. Start UnDieting**
Stop yo-yo dieting and stop following a diet plan.

☐ **#2. Start one change per week**
Implementing one action per week.

☐ **#3. Start doing it**
Set an action-oriented goal.

☐ **#4. Start using problem-solving techniques**
Look for ways to face your obstacles.

☐ **#5. Start your new life with a kick-off week**
Keep a food journal.

☐ **#6. Un-low**
Skip low-sugar or low-fat products.

☐ **#7. Un-shun boxes**
Cut out the worst HPF offenders!

☐ **#8. Un-cartoon**
Avoid products with cartoon characters on the box.

☐ **#9. Un-fat-free**
Fat-free food is not real food!

☐ **#10. Un-panel**
Check both the Nutrition Facts panel and the ingredients list.

☐ **#11. Un-miss partially hydrogenated oil**
Skip products with partially hydrogenated oil.

☐ **#12. Un-HPF**
Instead of focusing on how much meat or how many eggs you've eaten this week, channel that energy to the HPF instead.

☐ **#13. Un-plant omega-3**
Do not waste money getting plant-sourced ALA.

☐ **#14. Un-nitpick your cooking oil**
Stock a few good cooking oils at home.

☐ **#15. Un-palm**
Remember, no solid fats are good.

☐ **#16. Un-favor whole grain logos**
A whole grain claim on the front package does not mean a product is 100% whole grain.

☐ **#17. Uncover whole**
Look for the word "whole" in the ingredients list.

☐ **#18. Unleash whole grains from breakfast**
Don't limit your whole grains to breakfast.

☐ **#19. Un-expect benefits from isolated fiber**
Skip HPF with added fiber.

☐ **#20. Un-halt your grains; let them sprout**
Try sprouted grains for a softer texture with all the benefits of whole grains.

☐ **#21. Be unafraid of meat**
It's not as high in fat or calories as many junk foods!

☐ **#22. Un-medicate your meat**
Choose meat from animals that are raised naturally.

☐ **#23. Un-crate eggs**
Eggs don't increase blood cholesterol or lead to weight gain.

☐ **#24. Unveil fish**
Not all fish is high in mercury.

☐ **#25. Undo your relationship with processed meat**
Processed meats should simply be avoided.

☐ **#26. Un-drink your calories**
Drinks are meant to hydrate us, not feed us, so they shouldn't be a big source of calories.

☐ **#27. Un-medicate your milk**
Buy organic whenever possible.

☐ **#28. Understand the UnDiet formula: 3+1**
Drink three calcium-containing drinks per day (dairy or non-dairy) and have only one discretionary drink.

☐ **#29. Un-super-size your discretionary drinks**
A serving is eight ounces.

☐ **#30. Un-bore your water**
Jazz up water with a tea bag or frozen fruit.

☐ **#31. Un-count 5-a-day and count 3-a-day instead**
Aim for three different colors of produce a day.

☐ **#32. Un-side your veggies**
Make your veggies a main dish.

☐ **#33. Un-complicate your beans**
Remember, beans are vegetables.

☐ **#34. Un-focus on fresh**
Frozen and canned produce offer the same nutritional benefits as the fresh stuff.

☐ **#35. Un-expense your organics budget**
You don't need to buy all-organic produce.

☐ **#36. Un-blame carbs and blame the extras instead**

☐ **#37. Un-dip finger foods**
Stop adding even more calories and fat by covering finger foods in sauces, dressings, and dips.

☐ **#38. Un-sweeten your drinks**
It's okay to add a couple teaspoons of sugar to your coffee, but don't go for drinks with loads of added sugar.

☐ **#39. Un-fake your sugar**
Instead of faking it with artificial sweeteners, slowly cut back on the amount of sugar you consume.

☐ **#40. Un-source your sugar**
All types of sugar have similar calorie levels.

□ **#41. Un-bank on yogurt to solve constipation**
Eat your yogurt as a dairy food, not a constipation remedy.

□ **#42. Un-complicate your breakfast cereal**
Stock a basic whole grain breakfast cereal as filler and mix it with others you love.

□ **#43. Un-soy-erize**
Eat natural soy foods, not fancy soy snacks.

□ **#44. Be un-swayed by fancy calcium marketing**
Focus on elemental calcium content when choosing a calcium supplement.

□ **#45. Un-generalize your multis**
Choose a multivitamin supplement that is gender-specific and age-specific.

□ **#46. Un-empty your calories**
Adding in a few nutrients does not make junk foods good for you.

□ **#47. Un-dashboard dine**
Mindful eating is an important factor in achieving your weight-loss goals.

□ **#48. Un-shun cooking**
A little bit of home cooking is better than none.

□ **#49. Unburden yourself**
Get help with shopping and cooking.

□ **#50. Un-count calories**
Eating healthy is not all about counting calories or grams of fat.

*For a printable version of these 50 Go UnDiet Actions at-a-glance, go to
http://www.healthcastle.com/GoUnDietActions*

About Gloria

Spreading the goodness of nutrition is Gloria's passion! She is committed to helping people lead healthier lifestyles through nutrition education and awareness. She is a veteran interview subject, and her articles regularly appear in national media, including *Reuters, FoxNews, NBC & ABC affiliates, iVillage*, and *USA Today*. Gloria is also regularly regarded as a nutrition expert and had been quoted in numerous publications such as *Women's Health, Women's Day, Chicago Sun-Times, Oxygen, Globe & Mail, National Post, Reader's Digest, Today's Dietitian*, and more.

Gloria is a member of the American Dietetic Association, Dietitians of Canada, and the College of Dietitians British Columbia. She has served as the Country Representative Chair for the American Overseas Dietetic Association (AODA) for two years. Gloria has also served on the National Advisory Committee of "Healthy Eating is in Store for You (HESY)"—a joint project developed by the Canadian Diabetes Association and Dietitians of Canada.

Gloria founded HealthCastle.com as a hobby site in 1997 when her father was diagnosed with cancer. Gloria began writing and compiling cancer nutrition articles for her family, and published them so that other families could benefit from the information as well.

Since then, the HealthCastle.com community has grown into a robust nutrition resource library featuring hundreds of articles, nutrition tools and calculators, exclusive nutrition guides, and a podcast. In 2008, HealthCastle.com officially became a USDA MyPyramid Corporate Partner, and in 2010, HealthCastle.com served over 7.5 million readers.

Connect with Gloria:

 facebook.com/HealthCastle

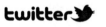 twitter.com/HealthCastleGlo

 GoUnDiet.com

Endnotes

[1] Shay LE, Seibert D, Watts D, Sbrocco T, Pagliara C. Adherence and weight loss outcomes associated with food-exercise diary preference in a military weight management program. Eat Behav. 2009 Dec;10(4):220–7. Epub 2009 Jul 16.

[2] O'Sullivan HL, Alexander, E, Ferriday D and Brunstrom JM. Effects of repeated exposure on liking for a reduced-energy-dense food. Am J Clin Nutr. 2010 Jun;91(6): 1584–9. Epub 2010 Apr 7.

[3] IOM (Institute of Medicine). Strategies to reduce sodium intake in the United States. Washington, DC: The National Academics Press; 2010.

[4] Hajjar IM, Grim CE, George V, Kotchen TA. Impact of diet on blood pressure and age-related changes in blood pressure in the US population. Arch Intern Med. 2001;161:589–593.

[5] Cook NR, Obarzanek E, Cutler JA, Buring JE, Rexrode KM, Kumanyika SK, et al. Joint effects of sodium and potassium intake on subsequent cardiovascular disease. Arch Intern Med. 2009;169(1):32–40.

[6] Fairfield H. Metrics: Factory food. The New York Times. 3 April 2010;Sect. BU:5. Print.

[7] Kellogg's® Froot Loops® cereal [Internet]. Kellogg NA Co.; c2010 [cited 2010 Apr 29]. Available from: http://www2.kelloggs.com/Product/ProductDetail.aspx?brand=153&product=566&cat=

[8] Oscar Mayer hot dogs – wieners – classic bun-length 8 ct [Internet]. Kraft Foods Inc.; c2010 [cited 2010 Jun 16]. Available from: http://www.kraftrecipes.com/Products/ProductInfoDisplay.aspx?SiteId=1&Product=4470000004

[9] General Mills: Brand product list page [Internet]. Minneapolis: General Mills; c2009 [cited 2010 Apr 28]. Available from: http://www.generalmills.com/corporate/brands/product_image.aspx?catID=23335&itemID=8854

[10] Oscar Mayer cold cuts – ham – smoked 96% fat free [Internet]. Kraft Foods Inc.; c2010 [cited 2010 Jun 16]. Available from: http://www.kraftrecipes.com/Products/ProductInfoDisplay.aspx?SiteId=1&Product=4470003014

[11] Kraft salad dressing – salad dressing – free Italian [Internet]. Kraft Foods Inc.; c2011 [cited 2011 Jan 18]. Available from: http://www.kraftrecipes.com/products/productinfodisplay.aspx?siteid=1&product=2100064271

[12] Otterman S. No brownies at bake sales, but Doritos may be O.K. 2010 Feb 23 [cited 2010 April 22]. In: The New York Times. City Room Blog [Internet]. New York: The New York Times Company c2010. Available from: http://cityroom.blogs.nytimes.com/2010/02/23/no-brownies-at-bake-sales-but-doritos-may-be-o-k/

[13] Doritos® Reduced Fat Cool Ranch® Flavored Tortilla Chips [Internet]. Frito-Lay North America, Inc.; c2011 [cited 2011 Jan 18]. Available from: http://www.fritolay.com/our-snacks/doritos-reduced-fat-cool-ranch.html

[14] Häagen-Dazs® | Products | Häagen-Dazs Five | Details: Milk Chocolate [Internet]. HDIP, Inc. [cited 2011 Jan 18]. Available from: http://www.haagen-dazs.com/ingredients/ingredient.aspx?id=370&name=milk+chocolate&seg=

[15] Horizon—Nutritional Facts—Ice Cream [Internet] [cited 2011 Jan 18]. Available from: http://www.horizondairy.com/ingredients/pop_nutri_ice_cream.html#ice_cream_chocolate

[16] Kraft salad dressing – salad dressing – light Caesar [Internet]. Kraft Foods Inc.; c2011 [cited 2011 Jan 18]. Available from: http://www.kraftfoods.com/kf/Products/ProductInfoDisplay.aspx?SiteId=1&Product=2100065474

[17] Rainer L, Heiss CJ. Conjugated linoleic acid: Health implications and effects on body composition. J Am Diet Assoc. 2004;104:963–8.

[18] Kris-Etherton P, Innis S. Position of the American Dietetic Association and Dietitians of Canada: Dietary fatty acids. J Am Diet Assoc. 2007;107:1599–1611.

[19] Kris-Etherton P, Yu S. Individual fatty acid effects on plasma lipids and lipoproteins: Human studies. Am J Clin Nut. 1997;65(suppl):1628S-1644S.

[20] Bonanaome A, Grundy S. Effect of dietary stearic acid on plasma cholesterol and lipoprotein levels. N Engl J Med. 1988;318:1244–8.

[21] MacLean CH, Newberry SJ, Mojica WA, Khanna P, Issa AM, Suttorp MJ, et al. Effects of omega-3 fatty acids on cancer risk: A systematic review. JAMA. 2006;295;403–15.

[22] Van Gelder BM, Tijhuis M, Kalmijn S, Kromhout D. Fish consumption, n-3 fatty acids, and subsequent 5-year cognitive decline in elderly men: The Zutphen Elderly Study. Am J Clin Nutr. 2007;85:1142–7.

[23] Gerster H. Can adults adequately convert alpha-linolenic acid (18:3 n-3) to eicosapentaenoic acid (20:5 n-3) and docosahexaenoic acid (22:6 n-3)? Int J Vitam Nutr Res. 1998;68(3):159–73.

[24] Brouwer IA, Katan MB, Zock PL. Dietary alpha-linolenic acid is associated with reduced risk of fatal coronary heart disease, but increased prostate cancer risk: A meta-analysis. J Nutr. 2004;134:919–22.

[25] Simon JA, Chen YH, Bent S. The relation of alpha-linolenic acid to the risk of prostate cancer: A systematic review and meta-analysis. Am J Clin Nutr. 2009;89(5):1558S-1564S.

[26] Hamazaki T, Okuyama H. The Japan Society for Lipid Nutrition recommends to reduce the intake of linoleic acid: A review and critique of the scientific evidence. World Rev Nutr Diet. 2003;92:109–32.

[27] International Society for the Study of Fatty Acids and Lipids. Recommendations for intake of polyunsaturated fatty acids in healthy adults. 2004 Jun.

[28] Pischon T, Hankinson SE, Hotamisligil GS, Rifai N, Willet WC, Rimm EB. Habitual dietary intake of n-3 and n-6 fatty acids in relation

to inflammatory markers among US men and women. Circulation. 2003;08:155–60.

[29] Garg A. High-monounsaturated-fat diets for patients with diabetes mellitus: A meta-analysis. Am J Clin Nutr. 1998;67(suppl):577S-582S.

[30] Chunky | Peanut Butter | Smucker's Products | Smucker's [Internet]. The J.M. Smucker Company [cited 2011 Jan 19]. Available from: http://www.smuckers.com/products/details.aspx?groupId=2&categoryId=11&flavorId=66

[31] Creamy Peanut Butter | Jif [Internet]. The J.M. Smucker Company [cited 2011 Jan 19]. Available from: http://www.jif.com/Products/Details?categoryId=64&productId=325

[32] National Cancer Institute. Usual Intake of Whole Grains [Internet]. National Cancer Institute Risk Factor Monitoring and Methods Branch Web site, Applied Research Program [updated 2010 April 13; cited 2010 April 27]. Available from: http://riskfactor.cancer.gov/diet/usualintakes/pop/t15.html

[33] Cheerios [Internet]. Minneapolis: General Mills; c2010 [cited 2011 Jan 19]. Available from: http://www.generalmills.com/~/media/Images/Brands/Nutritional_Images/Big_G/Cheerios-661.ashx

[34] Wonder Bread, Whole Grain, White [Internet]. Wegmans [cited 2011 Jan 19]. Available from: https://www.wegmans.com/webapp/wcs/stores/servlet/ProductDisplay?langId=-1&storeId=10052&productId=366403&catalogId=10002

[35] The Whole Grains Council. Identifying Whole Grain Products [Internet]. Oldways Preservation Trust/Whole Grains Council; c2003-07 [cited 2010 Apr 27]. Available from: http://www.wholegrainscouncil.org/whole-grains-101/identifying-whole-grain-products

[36] Slavin JL. Position of the American Dietetic Association: Health implications of dietary fiber. J Am Diet Assoc. 2009;109(2):350.

[37] American Dietetic Association. Position of the American Dietetic Association: Health implications of dietary fiber. J Am Diet Asso. 2008;108:1716–1731.

[38] Chavan JK, Kadam SS. Nutritional improvement of cereals by sprouting. Critical Reviews in Food Science and Nutrition. 1989;28(5):401–37.

[39] Ito Y, Mizukuchi A, Kise M, Aoto H, Yamamoto S, Yoshihara R, et al. Postprandial blood glucose and insulin responses to pre-germinated brown rice in healthy subjects. J Med Invest. 2005 Aug;52:159–64.

[40] Hsu TF, Kise M, Wang MF, Ito Y, Yang MD, Aoto H, et al. Health benefits: Pre-germinated brown rice favorably affected fasting blood glucose, fructosamine, serum total cholesterol, and triacylglycerol levels in human subjects. J Nutr Sci Vitaminol (Tokyo). 2008 Apr;54(2):163–8.

[41] Powell, BA. Breaking news: USDA limits "grass fed" label to meat that actually is. 2007 Oct 16 [cited 2010 May 13]. In: The Ethicurean [Internet]. Available from: http://www.ethicurean.com/2007/10/16/grass-fed-label/

[42] Daley CA, Abbott A, Doyle PS, Nader GA, and Larson S. A review of fatty acid profiles and antioxidant content in grass-fed and grain-fed beef. Nut Jour 2010;9:10.

[43] Acevedo N, Lawrence JD, and Smith M. Organic, Natural and Grass-Fed Beef: Profitability and constraints to Production in the Midwestern U.S. [Internet]. Iowa State University; 2006 [cited 2010 May 13]. Available from: http://www.iowabeefcenter.org/content/Organic_Natural_Grass_Fed_Beef_2006.pdf

[44] Humane Society of the United States. Meat and Dairy Labels: A brief guide to labels and animal welfare [Internet]. The Society; c2010 [updated 2009 Nov 9; cited 2010 May 13]. Available from: http://www.humane society.org/issues/confinement_farm/facts/meat_dairy_labels.html

[45] Li H, Stampfer MJ, Giovannucci EL, et al. A prospective study of plasma selenium levels and prostate cancer risk. J Natl Cancer Inst. 2004;96(9):696–703.

[46] U.S. Food and Drug Administration. Mercury Levels in Commercial Fish and Shellfish [Internet]. U.S. Department of Health and Human Services [updated 2009 Nov 11; cited 2010 May 10]. Available from: http://www.fda.gov/Food/FoodSafety/Product-SpecificInformation/Seafood/FoodbornePathogensContaminants/Methylmercury/ucm115644.htm

[47] Natural Resources Defense Council. Mercury Contamination in Fish [Internet]. The Council [cited 2010 May 10]. Available from: http://www.nrdc.org/health/effects/mercury/guide.asp

[48] Food and Nutrition Board, Institute of Medicine. Seafood choices: Balancing benefits and risk. Washington, DC: National Academies Press; 2007.

[49] World Cancer Research Fund/American Institute for Cancer Research. Food, nutrition, physical activity, and the prevention of cancer: A global perspective. Washington, DC: AICR; 2007.

[50] Cross AJ, Ferrucci LM, Risch A, et al. A large prospective study of meat consumption and colorectal cancer risk: An investigation of potential mechanisms underlying this association. Cancer Research. 2010;70:2406–14.

[51] Popkin BM. Patterns of beverage use across the lifecycle. Physiol Behav. 2010;100(1):4–9.

[52] Johnson RK et al. for the American Heart Association Nutrition Committee of the Council on Nutrition, Physical Activity and Metabolism and the Council on Epidemiology and Prevention. Dietary sugars intake and cardiovascular health: A scientific statement from the American Heart Association. Circulation. 2009; 120:1011–20.

[53] Centers for Disease Control and Prevention, National Health and Nutrition Examination Survey 2005–2006.

[54] Lipton Iced Tea with Lemon Flavor [Internet]. Unilever; c2011 [cited 2010 May 22]. Available from http://www.liptont.com/our_products/iced_tea/ice_lemon.aspx

[55] Suter PM and Trembaly A. Is alcohol consumption a risk factor for weight gain and obesity? Crit Rev Clin Lab Sci. 2005;42(3):197–227.

[56] Keast D et al. Contributions of milk, dairy products, and other foods to vitamin D intakes in the U.S.: NHANES, 2003–2006. FASEB J. 24:745.9.

57 Brehm BJ, D'Alessio DA. Benefits of high-protein weight loss diets: Enough evidence for practice? Curr Opin Endocrinol Diab Obes. 2008.15(5):416–21.

58 Clifton P. The science behind weight loss diets—a brief review. Aust Fam Physician. 2006;35(8):580–2.

59 Garavello W, Giordano L, Bosetti C, Talamini R, Negri E, Tavani A, et al. Diet diversity and the risk of oral and pharyngeal cancer. Eur J Nutr. 2008;47(5):280–4.

60 National Cancer Institute. Usual Intake of Cooked Dry Beans & Peas [Internet]. National Cancer Institute Risk Factor Monitoring and Methods Branch Web site, Applied Research Program [updated 2010 Apr 13; cited 2010 May 5]. Available from: http://riskfactor.cancer.gov/diet/usualintakes/pop/t7.html

61 Organic Trade Association. U.S. Organic Product Sales Reach $26.6 Billion in 2009 [Internet]. The Association; 2010 [updated 2010 Apr 22; cited 2010 May 6]. Available from: http://www.organicnewsroom.com/2010/04/us_organic_product_sales_reach_1.html

62 Lairon D. 2009. Nutritional quality and safety of organic food. A review. Agron Sustain Dev. 2010;30:33–41. Epub 2009 Jul 8.

63 Dangour AD, Dodhia SK, Hayter A, Allen E, Lock K, and Uauy R. Nutritional quality of organic foods: a systematic review. J Clin Nutr. 2009 Sep; 90(3):680–5. Epub 2009 Jul 29.

64 Gibson S. Sugar-sweetened soft drinks and obesity: a systematic review of the evidence from observational studies and interventions. Nutr Res Rev. 2008;21(2)134–47.

65 Stookey JD, Constant F, Gardner CD, Popkin BM. Replacing sweetened caloric beverages with drinking water is associated with lower energy intake. Obesity (Silver Spring). 2007 Dec;15(12):3013–22.

66 Malik VS, Schulze MB, Hu FB. Intake of sugar-sweetened beverages and weight gain: A systematic review. Am J Clin Nutr. 2006;84:274–88.

[67] Mattes RD, Popkin BM. Nonnutritive sweetener consumption in humans: Effects on appetite and food intake and their putative mechanisms. Am J Clin Nutr. 2009 Jan;89(1):1–14.

[68] Dhingra R, Sullivan L, Jacques PF, et al. Soft drink consumption and risk of developing cardiometabolic risk factors and the metabolic syndrome in middle-aged adults in the community. Circulation. 2007;116:480–8.

[69] Swithers SE, Baker CR, Davidson TL. General and persistent effects of high-intensity sweeteners on body weight gain and caloric compensation in rats. Behav Neurosci. 2009 Aug;123(4):772–80.

[70] Brown RJ, de Banate MA, Rother KI. Artificial sweeteners: A systematic review of metabolic effects in youth. Int J Pediatr Obes. 2010 Aug;5(4):305–12. Epub 2010 Jan 18.

[71] Mattes RD and Popkin BM. Nonnutritive sweetener consumption in humans: Effects on appetite and food intake and their putative mechanisms. Am J Clin Nutr. 2009;289:1–14.

[72] Pepsi Product Information: Pepsi [Internet] [cited 2011 Jan 20]. Available from: http://www.pepsiproductfacts.com/infobyproduct.php

[73] Cheerios [Internet]. General Mills. [cited 2011 Jan 20] Available from: http://www.cheerios.com/ourcereals/ourcereals_home.aspx

[74] Benecol [Internet]. Ft. Washington, PA: McNeil Nutritionals, LLC; c2002-11 [cited 2011 Jan 21]. Available from: http://benecolusa.com/products/index.jhtml?id=benecol/products/spreadFacts.inc

[75] Sacks FM, Lichtenstein A, Van Horn L, Harris W, Kris-Etherton P, and Winston M for the American Heart Association Nutrition Committee. Soy protein, isoflavones, and cardiovascular health: An American Heart Association science advisory for professionals from the Nutrition Committee. Circulation. 2006;113:1034–44.

[76] Erdman JW, Badger TM, Lampe JW, Setchell KDR, and Messina M. Not all soy products are created equal: Caution needed in interpretation of research results. J Nutr. 2004;134:1229S-1233S.

[77] Ervin RB, Wright JD, Wang CY, Kennedy-Stephenson J. Dietary intake of selected vitamins for the United States population: 199–2000. National Center for Health Statistics Advance Data 339. 2004 Mar 12.

[78] Miller ER, Pastor-Barriuso R, Dala D, Riemersma RA, Appel LJ, Gullar E. Meta-analysis: High dose vitamin E supplementation may increase all-cause mortality. Ann Intern Med. 2005;142:37–46.

[79] Bairati I, Meyer F, Gélinas M, Fortin A, Nabid A, Brochet F, et al. A randomized trial of antioxidant vitamins to prevent second primary cancers in head and neck cancer patients. J Natl Cancer Inst. 2005 Apr 6;97(7):481–8.

[80] Epstein LH, Gordy CC, Raynor HA, Beddome M, Kilanowski CK, Paluch R. Increasing fruit and vegetable intake and decreasing fat and sugar intake in families at risk for childhood obesity. Obesity Res 2001;9(3):171–8.

[81] Epstein LH, Raluch RA, Beecher MD, Roemmich JN. Increasing healthy eating vs. reducing high energy-dense foods to treat pediatric obesity. Obesity (Silver Spring) 2008;16(2):318–26.

[82] Larson NI, Nelson MC, Neumark-Sztainer D, Story M, Hannan PJ. Making time for meals: Meal structure and associations with dietary intake in young adults. J Am Diet Assoc. 2009 Jan;109(1):72–9.

[83] Mathieu J. What should you know about mindful and intuitive eating? J Am Diet Assoc. 2009 Dec;109(12):1982–7.

[84] Rodriguez LM, Castellanos VM. Use of low-fat foods by people with diabetes decreases fat, saturated fat, and cholesterol intakes. J Am Diet Assoc. 2000;100(5):531–6.

[85] U.S. Department of Agriculture. MyPyramid Food Intake Patterns [Internet]. USDA; 2005 [cited 2011 Jan 4]. Available from: http://www.mypyramid.gov/downloads/MyPyramid_Food_Intake_Patterns.pdf

Index

Page numbers followed by (t)
indicate a table.

A

acesulfame-potassium (Ace-K), 15,
    125
aging and supplements, 142
ALA, 37–38
    See also omega-3 fats
alcohol, 87–90, 149
    See also specific types of alcohol
algae oil, 144
allicin, 105
amino acids, essential, 56
anthocyanins, 104, 105
anthoxanthins, 105
antibiotics, 92
antioxidants, 103, 136
    *See also specific types of
        antioxidants*
artificial sweeteners, 15, 62,
    125–126, 125(t)
Asian noodles, 57
aspartame, 15, 125

B

barley, 55
beans, 108–110
beer, 88
beta-carotenes, 105, 115, 142
    See also vitamin A
Bifidus regularis, 132
Bifodobacterium lactis, 132
birth defects, 143, 144
bloating/gas, 62–63
blood clotting/coagulation, 50, 88
blood pressure, 16–17, 50, 105,
    125–126, 162
blood sugar/glucose, 48, 59, 159
    See also diabetes
bone mineral density, 144
    See also osteoporosis
breakfast cereal, 133–134
brown rice, 56
brown rice noodles, 57
bulgur, 56

C

cage-free chicken, 69

cage-free eggs, 71
calcium, 59, 93–95, 143–144, 160
calorie calculator (website), 68, 164
calories
    in alcohol, 88
    carbs vs. protein, 100–101,
        100–101(t)
    counting, 155–156
    cutting, 2–3
    defined, 2
    in dips, dressings, and sauces,
        120–121, 120–121(t)
    low fat foods, 13–14, 156
    in meat, 65–66, 66(t)
    negative calorie balance, 9
    in processed meats, 80–81(t)
    in regular and reduced-fat
        foods, 14(t)
    in seafood and meat, 73–74(t)
    in snack foods, 67(t)
    in sugar, 129, 129(t)
    in sugar-sweetened drinks,
        85(t), 161
Canadian dairy products and
    growth hormones, 93
cancer
    ALA and, 37
    alcohol and, 88
    allicin and, 105
    anthocyanins and, 104, 105
    beta-carotenes and, 105
    CLA and, 34
    colorful foods and, 103
    fiber and, 48, 59, 159
    fish and, 37
    lycopene and, 104
    omega-6 fats and, 38
    processed meats and, 79, 81

selenium and, 74
sulforaphane and, 104
trans fats and, 32
vitamin D and, 142, 160
vitamin E and, 145
whole grains and, 50
carbs (carbohydrates), 99–101,
    100–101(t), 118–119, 119(t)
cartoon characters, 23–24
central nervous system disorders,
    144–145
certified humane animal husbandry,
    69
cheese, 122, 132
chemicals in processed foods, 22
cholesterol
    breakfast cereal and, 133–134
    dietary vs. blood, 72
    eggs and, 72–73
    fiber and, 48, 59, 159
    grass-fed beef and, 68
    margarine-style spreads and,
        135–136
    omega-3 fats and, 36, 137
    omega-6 fats and, 39
    psyllium and, 134
    resveratrol and, 88
    saturated fat and, 34
    soda/diet soda and, 125
    soluble fiber and, 59
    soy and, 138–139
    stearic acid and, 34
    whole grains and, 50
    See also HDL cholesterol;
        LDL cholesterol
CLA (conjugated linoleic acid), 34
coagulation/blood clotting, 50, 88
cocktails/coolers, 89–90

coconut oil, 34, 44–45
cognitive decline, 37
colorful fruits and vegetables, 103–105
colorings in processed foods, 21
common whole grains, 49(t)
community-supported agriculture (CSA), 115
conjugated linoleic acid (CLA), 34
constipation, 48, 59, 131–133, 145
cooking, 106–107, 151–154, 160–161
cooking oils, 40–45, 42(t)
coolers/cocktails, 89–90
CSA (community-supported agriculture), 115
cystic fibrosis, 45

D
DHA, 37–38, 74, 137, 144
    See also omega-3 fats
diabetes, 15, 32, 48, 50, 59, 159
diarrhea, 131
diet fatigue, 1
diet plans, 2–3, 163
diet soda/soda, 87, 95, 124–127, 130, 161
dips, calories in, 120–121, 120–121(t)
Dirty Dozen (pesticide worst offenders), 114
diverticulosis, 48
dressings, calories in, 120–121, 120–121(t)
drinks
    calorie intake from, 85
    calories in sugar-sweetened, 85(t), 161
    consumption patterns, 84–85

and rehydration, 86
serving size, 95–96
sugar in, 124
super size, 96(t)
UnDiet Formula: 3+1, 93–94
    See also alcohol; milk; tea

E
eating decisions, conscious, 150–151
eating on the run, 150–151
eggs, 71–73
elemental calcium, 144
empty-calorie foods, 148–150, 149(t)
EPA, 37–38, 136–137
    See also omega-3 fats
essential amino acids, 56
essential fatty acids, 74
excuses/obstacles, 5–7
exercise, 9
exotic fruit juices, 136

F
families, cooking together, 154
farmers markets, 114
fat
    in meat, 65–66, 66(t)
    in processed meats, 80–81(t)
    in regular and reduced-fat foods, 14(t)
    in seafood and meat, 73–74(t)
    in snack foods, 67(t)
fat-free food, 24–25
fats
    bad fats, 31–36
    cooking oils, 40–45, 42(t)
    good fats, 36–40
    monounsaturated fats, 34
    neutral fats, 35, 39

nut butters, 45–46
omega-3 fats, 36–38,
    136–137, 144
omega-6 fats, 38–39
omega-9 fats, 34, 39–40
saturated fats, 34–35, 162–163
trans fats, 32–34, 72–73
tropical plant oils, 34, 35,
    43–45
fatty acids, essential, 74
fatty acids, monounsaturated
  See omega-9 fats
fatty acids, poly-unsaturated, 139
fiber, 48–49, 58–61, 61(t), 133–134,
    159
50 small actions to undiet, 171–175
fish oil/DHA supplements, 38
fish/seafood, 38, 73–74(t), 73–79
5-Second Scan
    cartoon characters, 23–24
    fat-free food, 24–25
    nutrition facts and ingredients
        list, 25–27
flavonoid phenolics, 87–88
flavonoids, 88
flaxseed oil, 37–38
folic acid/folate, 104, 142–143
food, growing, 115–116
food groups, requirements, 165
food journaling, 7–8
food labels, 32–34, 51, 68–69, 138
foods to eat less of, 161–163
foods to eat more of, 159–161
forbidden foods and guilt, 155–156
free radicals, 74
free-range eggs, 71
free-range poultry, 69
free-run chicken, 69

free-run eggs, 71
frozen/canned vegetables, 110–112
frozen fruit ice cubes, 97
fructose, 127
  See also sugar
fruit juices, exotic, 136
fruits/vegetables, 102–105, 102(t),
    104–105(t), 146
  See also vegetables
functional foods, 131

G
gardening, 115–116
gas/bloating, 62–63
gastrointestinal diseases, 45
glucose/blood sugar, 48, 59, 159
  See also diabetes
glycemic index (GI), 128
Go UnDiet Actions, 171–175
goat's milk, 91–92
good foods vs. bad foods, 155–156
grass-fed beef, 68
growing food, 115–116
growth hormones, 90–93

H
habits, establishing, 4–5
HDL cholesterol, 36–37, 88
  See also cholesterol
HealthCastle.com, 177
heart disease
    anthocyanins and, 104
    beta carotenes and, 105
    breakfast cereal and, 133
    CLA and, 34
    eggs and, 72–73
    fiber and, 48, 59
    folate and, 104

iron and, 145
lutein, 104
margarine-style spreads
    and, 135
omega-6 fats and, 38
plant sterols and, 135
seafood and, 74
sodium and, 162
sodium/potassium ratio
    and, 17
soy and, 138
trans fats and, 32
whole grains and, 50
hemorrhoids, 48
HFCS (high fructose corn syrup),
    127
high blood pressure, 16, 17, 162
high fructose corn syrup (HFCS),
    127
highly processed foods (HPF)
    avoiding/cutting back, 28–29,
        36, 40
    chemicals, colorings, and
        preservatives in, 21–22
    coconut/palm oils and, 34–35,
        42–45
    low fat/low sugar (the "low"
        road), 13–17
    and meat compared, 67
    partially hydrogenated oil in, 33
    saturated fats in, 35
    sodium in, 22–23, 162
    as weakest link, 148
    worst offenders, 20–26
home cooking, 151–154
hormone-free beef/milk, 69
HPF See highly processed foods
    (HPF)

hunger and artificial sweeteners,
    126
hunger cues, 151
hypertension See high blood
    pressure

I
immune function, 74, 105
inflammation, 38
ingredients lists, 26–27, 52–54
insoluble fiber, 58–61
intestinal pH, 59
iron, 145
isoflavones, 138
isolated fiber, 59–60

K
kidney-related health problems, 18
kosher salt, 16

L
L. bulgaricus, 131–132
L. casei immunitas, 132, 133
labeling loopholes, 33
lactase, 62
lactose intolerance, 62, 91, 132
lauric acid, 34
LDL cholesterol
    fiber and, 48, 159
    omega-3 fats and, 36, 137
    omega-6 fats and, 38–39
    soluble fiber and, 59
    soy and, 138
    stearic acid and, 34
    See also cholesterol
legumes See beans
lentils See beans
linoleic acid, 39

liquors/liqueurs, 90

listeria/listeriosis, 79, 81–82

liver abnormalities, and vitamin A, 144

LocalHarvest.org/csa, 115, 155

low-fat foods and calories, 13–14, 156

low-sugar foods/artificial sweeteners, 15

lutein, 104

lycopene, 104

M

macular degeneration, 104

maltitol, 62

margarine-style spreads, 135–136

marine-based vs. plant-based omega 3 fats, 37–38, 136–137, 144

meat, 65–69, 66(t), 70t, 73–74(t), 79–82

Mediterranean diet, 39

medium-chained triglycerides (MCT), 45

mercury in seafood, 74–79, 75–77(t)

metabolic syndrome, 125–126

micro-algae, 37

milk, 90–95

millet, 55–56

mindful eating, 150–151

monounsaturated fatty acids (MUFA) See omega-9 fats

MUFA (monounsaturated fatty acids) See omega-9 fats

multivitamins, 144

MyPyramid dietary guidelines, 108

myristic acid, 34

N

natural sugar, 128

natural/naturally raised livestock, 69

negative calorie balance, 9

neotame, 15, 125

neural tube defects, 143

neutral fats, 35, 39

nitrates/nitrites, 79

No More Packaged Foods (website), 153–154

non-dairy milk, 92

nut butters, 45–46

nuts, 19, 39–40, 45–46, 61, 101, 170

nutrition facts/ingredients list, 25–27

nutrition requirements, 164

O

oats, 49, 51, 54, 59, 169

obesity, 15, 158

obstacles/excuses, 5–7

oils, cooking, 40–45

omega-3 fats, 36–38, 136–137, 144

omega-3 fortified foods, 37, 71, 136–137

omega-6 fats, 38–39

omega-6/omega-3 ratio, 39

omega-9 fats, 34, 39–40

orange juice, 94

organic
    eggs, 71–72
    fruits and vegetables, 112–116
    meat, 68, 70
    milk, 91–93

osteoporosis, 142, 160

overeating, 20, 118, 126, 161

P

packaged foods *See* processed foods

palm oil, 34, 43–44

palmitic acid, 34

partially hydrogenated oil, 32–33
  See also trans fats

plant sterols, 135

plant-based vs. marine-based omega
  3 fats, 37–38, 136–137, 144

poly-unsaturated fatty acids, 139

popcorn, 58

potassium, 17–18, 18(t), 160

pregnancy, 142–143

preservatives in processed foods, 21

probiotics, 132

processed eggs, 72

processed foods, 11–13, 18–19
  See also highly processed foods
  (HPF)

processed meats, 79–82, 80–81(t)

psyllium, 134

pulses *See* beans

Q

quinoa, 56

R

resveratrol, 88

rigid meal plans, 2–3, 163

rules for eating, 155–156

S

S. thermophilus, 131–132

saccharin, 15, 125

salt *See* sodium

saturated fat in seafood and meat,
  73–74(t)

saturated fats, 34–35, 162–163

sauces, calories in, 120–121,
  120–121(t)

sea salt, 16

seafood/fish, 38, 73–74(t), 73–79

seeds, 40, 59, 61, 106, 169–170

selenium, 45, 74

smoking, 142–143

snack foods, calories, fat, and sugar
  in, 67(t)

snacks, 20, 166–168

soba, 57

soda/diet soda, 87, 95, 124–127,
  130, 161

sodium, 15–17, 22–23, 62, 80–81(t),
  162

sodium-to-potassium ratio, 17

soluble fiber, 58–61, 133–134

sorbitol, 62

soy, 138–139

spina bifida., 143

sprouted grains, 61, 63

stearic acid, 34

sterols, plant, 135

steviol glycosides, 125

stomach acid, 142

sucralose, 15, 125

sugar, 67(t), 122–124, 123(t),
  128–129, 129(t), 161

sugar alcohols, 62

sugar substitutes, 15, 62, 125–
  126, 125(t) *See also* artificial
  sweeteners

sulforaphane, 104

sunscreen, 141–142, 160

super foods, 169–170

supplements/vitamins, 141–146

sustainable seafood lists, 78

T

30 snacks under 200 calories,
166–168
tea, 86–87
textured vegetable (or soy) protein,
138
thyroid function, 74
toppings, 118–119
total fat and saturated fat content,
35(t)
trans fats, 32–34, 72–73
triglycerides, 36, 37, 88, 137
    See also medium-chained
        triglycerides (MCT)
tropical plant oils, 34, 35, 43–45

U

UnDiet formula: 3+1, 93–95

V

vaccenic acid, 34
vegetables, 105–107, 110–112
    See also fruits
vegetables, colorful, 103–105
villain foods, 9
vitamin A, 144–145

W

vitamin B12, 142
vitamin D, 141–142, 160
vitamin E, 145
vitamin water, 139, 140, 140(t)
vitamins/supplements, 141–146

W

water, 84–85, 96–97, 161
weakest link *See* highly processed
    foods (HPF)
weight gain, 9, 14, 88, 124, 126,
161
weight loss, 8, 39, 50, 99–100
wheat germ, 53
whole grains, 49–57
    See also specific types of whole
        grains
whole grains, recognizing, 54(t)
whole wheat udon, 57
wine, 87–89

X

xylitol, 62

Y

yogurt, 131–133

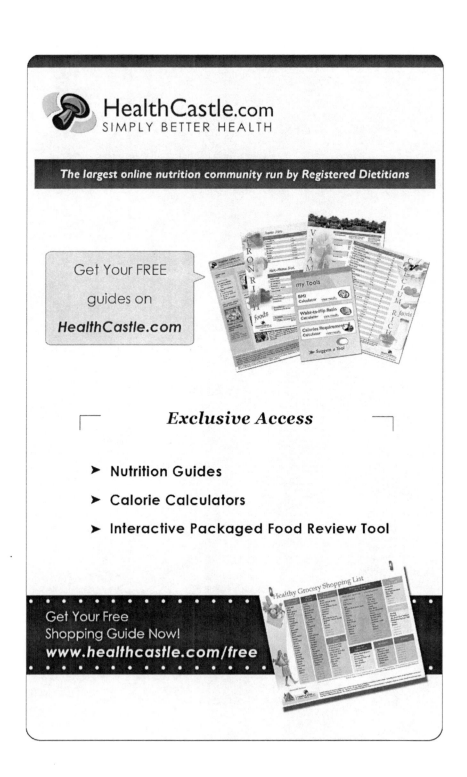

CPSIA information can be obtained at www.ICGtesting.com
Printed in the USA
LVOW090347080212

267650LV00008B/82/P